HEALTH AND SUCCESS

Active Learning Strategies to Promote Student Wellness

by Dorothy Michener

Incentive Publications, Inc.
Nashville, Tennessee

Illustrated by Gayle S. Harvey
Cover by Geoffrey Brittingham

ISBN 0-86530-412-2

Copyright © 1999 by Incentive Publications, Inc., Nashville, TN. All rights reserved. No part of this publication may be reproduced, stored in a retrieval system, or transmitted in any form or by any means (electronic, mechanical, photocopying, recording, or otherwise) without written permission from Incentive Publications, Inc., with the exception below.

Pages labeled with the statement **©1999 by Incentive Publications, Inc., Nashville, TN** are intended for reproduction. Permission is hereby granted to the purchaser of one copy of **HEALTH AND SUCCESS** to reproduce these pages in sufficient quantities for meeting the purchaser's own classroom needs.

PRINTED IN THE UNITED STATES OF AMERICA

Table of Contents

vii	**Preface**
9	**Chapter 1—Making the Right Choice**

Topics include
- peer pressure
- self-confidence
- decision making
- risk taking
- trust
- refusal skills
- assertiveness
- personal responsibility

21	**Chapter 2—Triple Trouble**

Topics include
- age-appropriate facts regarding substance abuse and prevention
- dependence
- addiction
- health hazards
- societal impact
- facing temptations

37	**Chapter 3—Help!**

Topics include
- potential risks
- self-help skills
- life-saving information regarding personal safety and violence prevention

49 | **Chapter 4—Big Changes, Big Choices**

Topics include
- sexuality
- dating
- fears
- facts
- AIDS concerns
- STD
- pregnancy

61 | **Chapter 5—The Need to Know**

Topics include
- teen suicide
- living with terminal illness
- handicapping conditions
- family pressures
- stress
- depression

73 | **Chapter 6—Natural Awakenings**

Topics include
- positive approaches to good health and wellness
- improving the quality of life—physically
- mental health
- emotional health

91 | **Appendix—Briefly**
— Marijuana alert
— Health Briefs
— Don't Go To Pot
— Getting to Know You
— Getting Help

PREFACE

The twentieth century has been called the Age of Anxiety . . . the Century of Stress.

The following six chapters focus on getting in touch—body and mind. Real and imaginary situations are presented about which to think. Some subject matters are more personal than others and teachers are encouraged to be sensitive as they talk with students.

Teachable Moments
    Activities in this book may be used at any time, without sequence. However, the most effective time would follow a similar curriculum topic or school "happening." Timely events in the media can often lead to class discussion and worksheet follow-up. Teachable moments are unpredictable and can pop up at any time.

Cross-Age Teaching
    Some of the student worksheets are appropriate for older students to use with younger ones. Activities on peer pressure and learning to "say no" are most effective when presented by slightly older mentors.

Bloom's Taxonomy
    The thinking process begins with knowledge and progresses to evaluation, and ideas. The work pages in this book fit into Benjamin Bloom's Taxonomy of Educational Objectives:

        Knowledge = Identifying;

        Comprehension = Understanding;

        Application = Applying the understandings;

        Analysis = Analyzing the qualities;

        Synthesis = Creating;

        Evaluation = Determining the effects/input of the qualities on self and society

The bulk of background information comes from your required curriculum (knowledge). The following pages provide more of the other taxonomy levels.

The News

The daily newspaper provides a good place to keep up with current health updates.

Adolescents are moving into a new age of exploration. For some it is an adventure, exciting and enriching; for others, adolescence is a time of fear as they encounter new feelings and vulnerability.

Today's youth are seldom carefree. Troubles can include drugs or alcohol, a dysfunctional family, abuse, school failure, terminal illness, sexuality, physical handicap, or the inability to cope. The problems that will not go away will cause stress. Physical health often will be affected when one is worried, fearful, or angry much of the time.

During the early adolescent years it is essential to urge kids to form a partnership—to work with the body and nourish the mind.

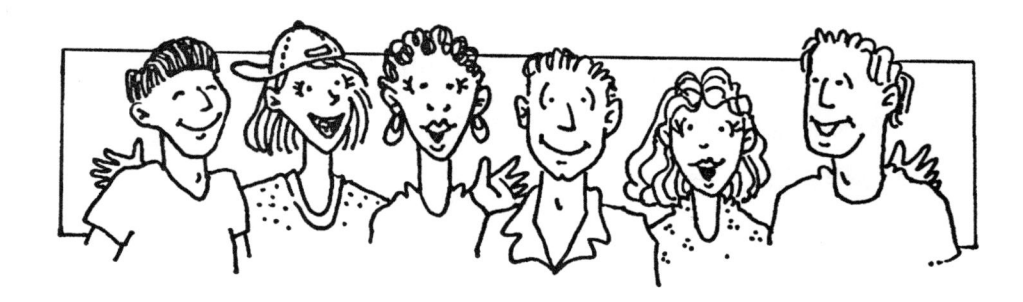

CHAPTER ONE

Making The Right Choice

10	**TEACHER'S PAGE**
11	*Everybody's Doing It!* Group "memberships"... What do they offer?
12	*The Out-Group* Ryan's scenario... What do you think?
13	*What's the Risk?* A risk and a hazard. How are they different?
14	*Keep Your Cool* Julie and Tracy's scenario... What do you think?
15	*Chicken* Where we get the term... Share your thoughts.
16	*The Compromise* Todd and Erika's scenario... What do you think?
17	*Pressure Points* Friend/family frictions... What can you do?
18	*Let's Pretend* An offer... How could I refuse?
19	*Getting Connected* Links between friends... What is really important?
20	*The "Muddle Plan"* A problem-solving strategy... It can work for you!

Health and Success

©1999 by Incentive Publications, Inc., Nashville, TN.

Making The Right Choice

With puberty comes a head-on rush into "junk" culture. It takes only a brief glance at a teen magazine to note that this time in a person's life can be both exciting and frightening. It's a risky world and one full of decisions and options.

One element of this world is peer-group pressure—an alarming phenomenon. Experience provides the ability to make prudent judgements and wise decisions. Young people, however, are anxious to please and to emulate their peers.

In this chapter we provide potentially dangerous scenarios in which a stand must be taken and a choice must be made.

Included in this chapter is an outline of a simple formula (the "muddle plan") to "de-fog" the brain, and enable it to work out the choices. The focus is on alternatives and consequences.

Although the first pages contain individual activities, sharing the completed work and discussing the outcomes is recommended. Self-confidence and an inner sense of focus should evolve.

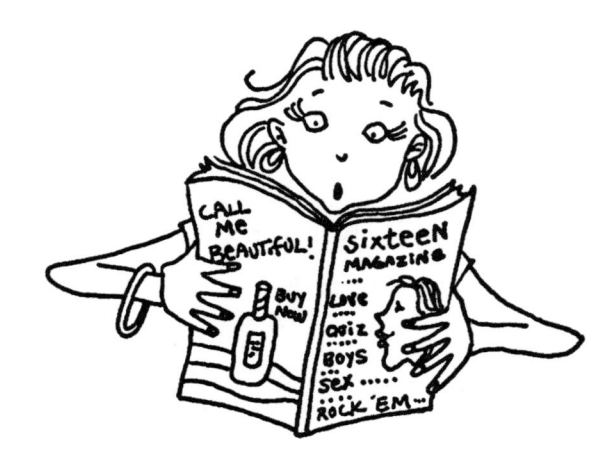

Everybody's Doing It!

SCENARIO

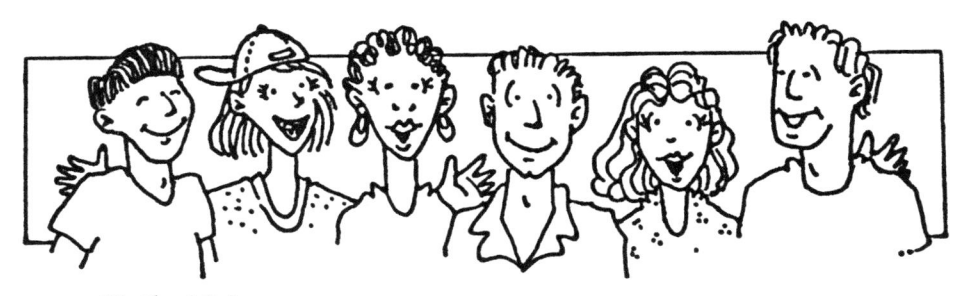

Group stuff, that is!

Sometimes kids pair up. Other times, it's fun to do things in one big group.

Your favorite group might be the hockey team, science club, or neighbors. Or, a group could be just classmates who enjoy being together. The reasons for different group membership change with time. What are your reasons today?

WRITE ABOUT IT

Most groups will fit into one of the following categories. Describe one or more groups you know of that meet your needs in these areas.

1. Common values

2. Friendship

3. Common interests

4. Similar intellect

5. Other

Focus Term: **Group** — *A number of persons or things considered, or ranged together that are related in some way.*

Health and Success

The Out Group

SCENARIO

Ryan is a learning-disabled twelve-year-old for whom school has always been a struggle. He has suffered years of embarrassment because he must leave his classmates to attend remedial programs. Often he is disruptive when he returns; he acts up and annoys others.

Ryan has been labeled a "trouble maker," and establishing long-term friendships is difficult for him. He does not fit into any of the school groups.

At one time, some older kids accepted him and offered to share their cigarettes and beer. Ryan refused and was quickly dropped by that group.

Ryan feels left out and is unhappy.

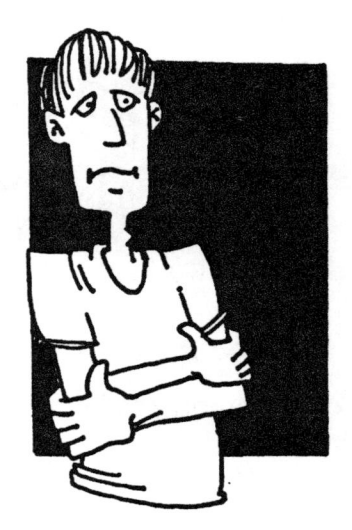

WHAT DO YOU THINK?

Is it important to belong to a group?

What do you think Ryan should do?

Can people still be happy when they are not part of a group?

What does Ryan's refusal to the older group tell you about him?

Focus Term: **Left Out** — Not included.

What's The Risk?

SCENARIO

Are "risks" and "hazards" the same?

Absolutely not!

A "hazard" is when people or the things they value are exposed to danger or harm. A "risk," however, is the measure of the likelihood of harm or loss that may come to you because of the hazard. A "risk" implies a threat of something that may happen.

Students your age are faced with countless hazards in everyday life. You are aware of most of them. It's important, however, to understand the risk involved when making a decision. Is it one worth taking?

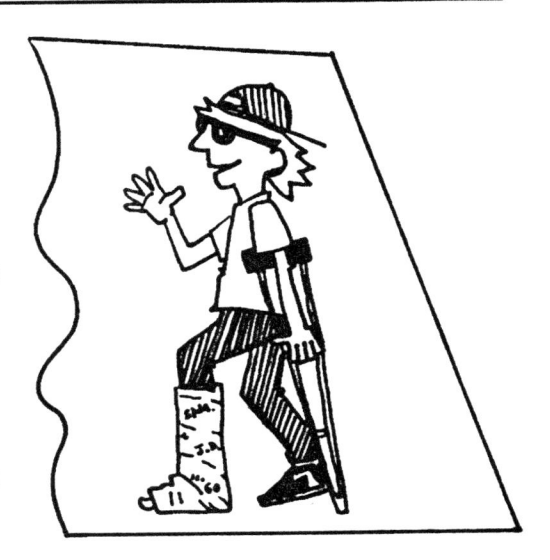

WHAT DO YOU THINK?

The following activities and technologies are thought to be risky by many people. Rank order their level of risk from one to twenty, according to how dangerous you think each to be.

What's the risk?

pesticides	hand guns	automobiles
fire fighting	flying in an airplane	drinking water
surfing	mountain climbing	auto racing
motorcycling	nuclear power	surgery
football	drinking alcohol	swimming
doing drugs	smoking	using firecrackers
policing	hang gliding	

Risk means different things to different people. Share your finished work with a classmate. Discuss the risks involved.

Focus Term: **Risk** — *Exposure to the chance of injury or loss.*

Keep Your Cool

SCENARIO

Julie and Tracy were thrilled to be invited to hang out after the game with some older kids. The girls felt proud to be seen with the popular group members. "We've arrived," said Julie. "We're cool!"

Later that evening they were offered some wine and a joint to smoke. Both girls refused, simply saying "No, thanks!"

At the end of the evening the two friends shared their feelings. They admitted that it was hard to say "no" because they were concerned about being ridiculed or shunned by the others.

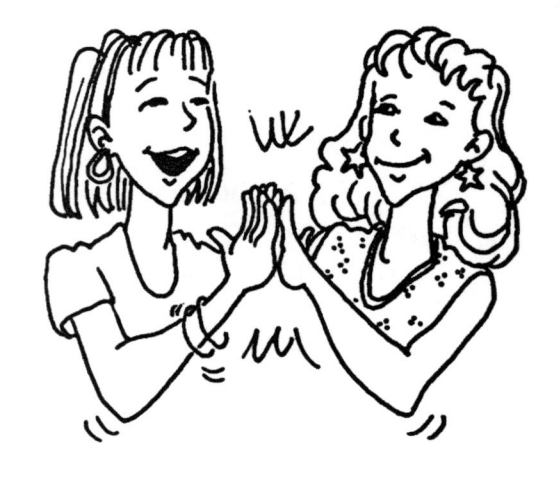

However, they laughed at what they called their "tryout." They decided that the popular group was not the group for them, and they felt good about their decision.

WHAT DO YOU THINK?

Have you had an experience when you were faced with a tough, peer-group decision? Write about it and how you kept or lost your cool. What are some ways to say "no"?

_____
_____
_____
_____
_____
_____
_____
_____
_____

Focus Term: **Ridicule** — *Words or actions aimed at contempt, deprecated.*

Chicken

SCENARIO

Have you ever wondered why people call you a "chicken" when you're afraid to do something? Why don't they say "you're a hippopotamus," or "you're a gorilla"?

Maybe it's because chickens scare easily and run away from danger.

Actually, chickens may have the right idea. They can't defend themselves very well, so why hang around? It's a matter of survival and that's smart!

Consider the risks and don't be afraid to say "no."

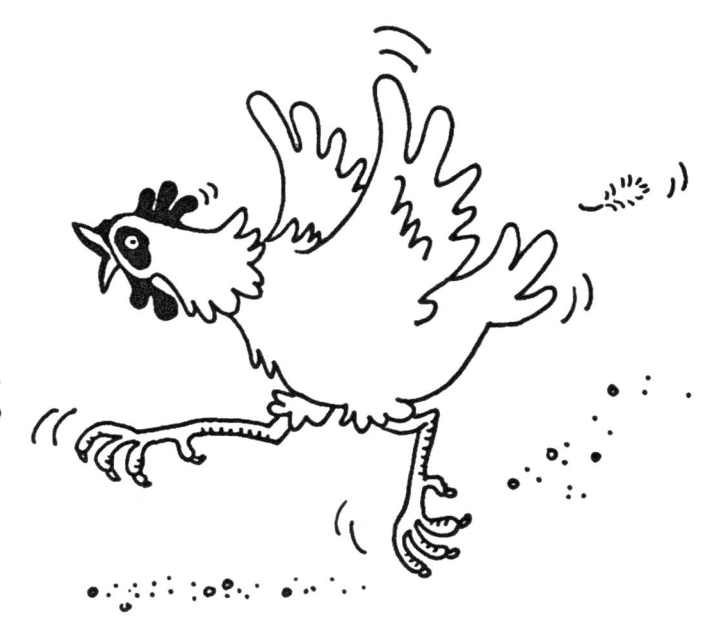

THOUGHTS TO SHARE

Have you ever been pressured to do something you did not want to do? What decision did you make? What else could you have done? How did you feel?

_____
_____
_____
_____
_____
_____
_____
_____
_____
_____

Focus Term: **Survival** — *To remain alive or intact after an event or occurrence.*

Health and Success

The Compromise

SCENARIO

Todd unexpectedly asked Erika to go to a party with him after the basketball game on Friday. She agreed excitedly, but on her way home she worried.

Although she was allowed to attend parties with a group, her parents said she was too young, at thirteen, to "date." She wondered—should she just go with Todd and tell her mom she was with the usual group? (The thought gave her an uncomfortable feeling.)

That evening, Erika and her mom discussed dating. Erika claimed that all her friends did it; her mom stood firm. However, after a lengthy discussion regarding the feelings of each, a compromise was reached.

Erika was allowed to go and meet Todd at the game, but she had to go to the party with a group of friends. It was OK if Todd was also at the party.

Erika had a great time at the game and at the party. She felt good about the compromise.

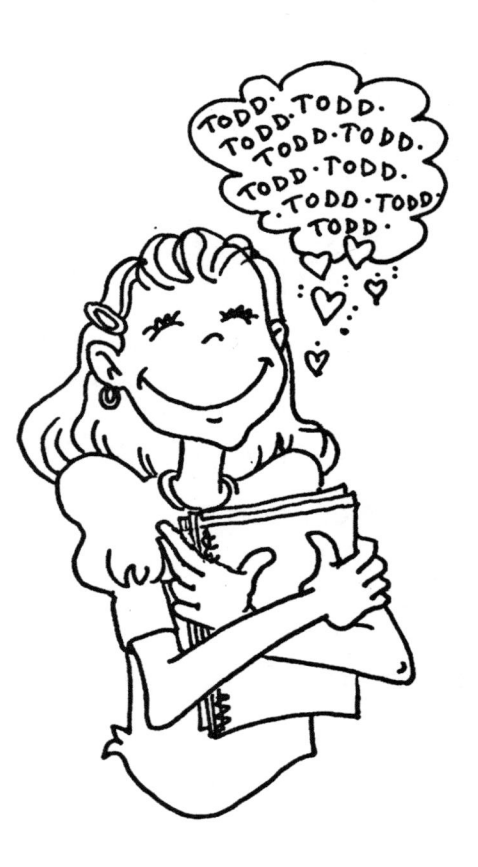

WHAT DO YOU THINK?

Learning to compromise takes patience, respect, and lots of honest communication. You negotiate for what you want, but don't always get it. A good compromise makes both individuals winners.

Have you ever worked out a compromise with a parent or friend? What happened? How did you feel? What did you learn?

Focus Term: **Compromise** — *A settlement of differences by mutual concessions.*

Pressure Points

SCENARIO

Does your group of friends sometimes want you to do things that, deep down, you really don't want to do?

Are there things your family is often on your case about? "Give me a break!" you might beg.

Friends want you to be like them. Your family is responsible for you. Often the two groups cause pressure in your life.

The following is a list of "pressure points." These are things about which parents and kids often disagree.

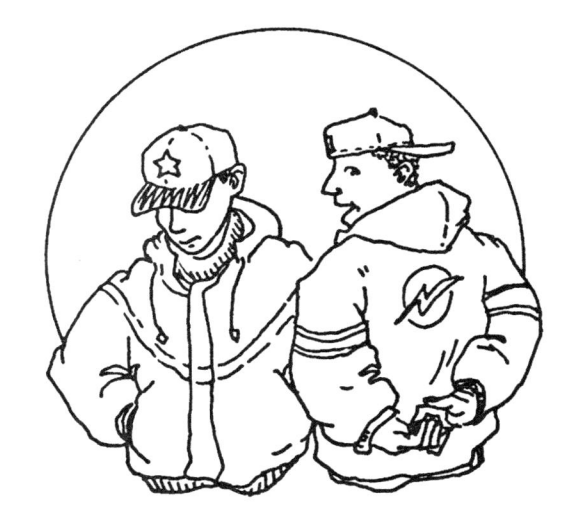

Look at the following list and check the issues that may cause problems in your life. Choose one to write about. How can you work it out?

clothing	dating	choice of friends
grades/homework	eating habits	movies/TV
wearing makeup	curfew	allowance
leisure time	responsibilities at home	substance abuse (smoking, drugs, alcohol).

This one is a problem: _____

WHAT CAN YOU DO ABOUT IT?

_____
_____
_____
_____
_____
_____

Focus Term: **Pressure** — *The exertion of a compelling force upon a person; harassment.*

Let's Pretend

SCENARIO

Let's pretend that you are feeling bored. Your best friend is away with his or her parents on vacation.

One day you get a phone call from someone you hardly know, who is in your math class. You are surprised and pleased to be invited to join the most popular kids in school for a weekend camp-out or a sleep-over party.

When you arrive, you find no adults present. Your new friends are smoking and drinking, and you are offered a can of beer. You have never used drugs and never want to. You feel strongly about your decision, but you don't want the other kids to make fun of you. Is this a clique you really care about?

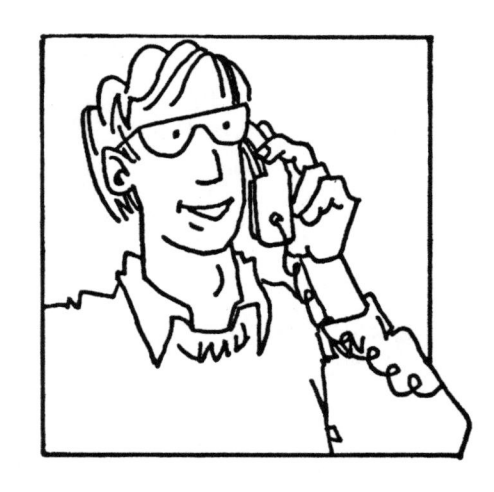

HOW COULD I REFUSE?

1. _____

2. _____

3. _____

4. _____

5. _____

Share your list with a classmate. Together, decide on the best response.

Getting Connected

SCENARIO

It's a struggle! Adolescence can be a period of great stress and turmoil. Those younger than you are thought to be "babies." Grown-up behavior is taboo. It's definitely confusing!

Having a close friend, or belonging to a group where you openly discuss things, can be important. Peers contribute to personal development and can influence behavior.

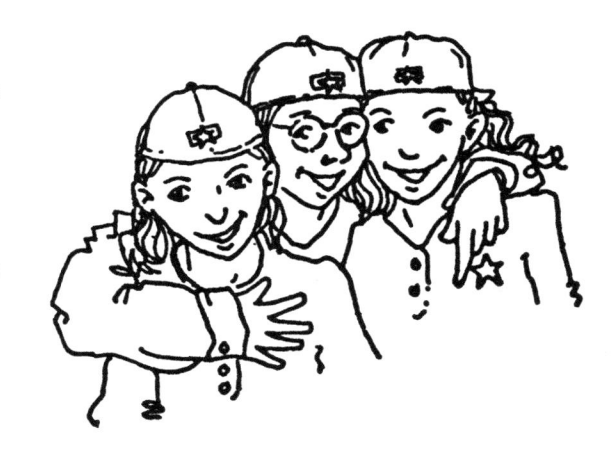

WHAT DO YOU THINK?

The following are thought to be important elements of friendship. Choose three you think are of high priority and explain your selections.

respect	**honesty**	**age**
fairness	**curiosity**	**intelligence**
acceptance	**adventure**	**race**
tolerance	**interests**	**same sex**

1. _____

2. _____

3. _____

Focus Term: **Adolescence** — *Growing into manhood or womanhood.*

The Muddle Plan

SCENARIO

Mark was having a hard time finding his way around the new middle school. It was confusing.

He did not know what to think of the kids in his classes. He felt unsure about one group that was very friendly, they asked him to hang out that weekend.

He decided to use his "muddle plan." It always helped when his brain felt muddled and fuzzy. This is what he does.

WHAT TO DO

1. Focus on what is happening

2. Pinpoint the problem

3. Learn more about it

4. Think of possible solutions

5. Consider the consequences (positive/negative)

6. Determine the best solution

The "muddle plan" helped Mark decide that this group would not make good friends, and he was right! That group got into big trouble that weekend and Mark was not involved.

Use the "muddle plan" to work out one of your problems.

Focus Term: **Muddle** — *Unable to think clearly.*

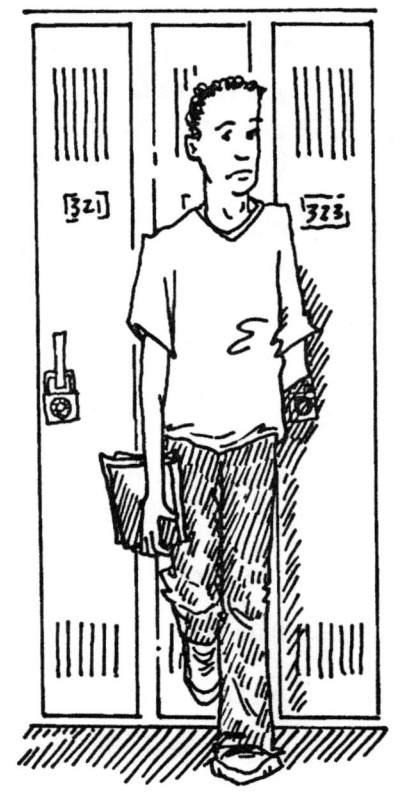

CHAPTER TWO

Triple Trouble

22	**TEACHER'S PAGE**
23	*A Clear Message* — Shannon's decision . . . What would yours be?
24	*Serious Business* — How drugs hurt . . . What do you know?
25	*Thoughts on Why* — Kids and drugs . . . What do you think?
26	*Joel's Story* — You decide . . . How will it end?
27	*Tips for Teens* — About marijuana . . . Did you know?
28	*More Tips for Teens* — About crack and cocaine . . . Did you also know?
29	*A Dangerous Chew* — Learn from the pros . . . Think and write.
30	*Chewed Out* — Let's imagine . . . What would you say?
31	*Smoke Rises* — Numbers increase . . . What can you do?
32	*Bad and Sad* — Robyn and Liz . . . What did they learn?
33	*About Alcohol* — Quick facts . . . Did you know?
34	*The Confrontation* — Think and write. How would you handle it?
35	*Hey! Put That Out* — You can save lives! Take action.
36	*Think Tank* — Bad habits . . . How can you stop?

Health and Success

©1999 by Incentive Publications, Inc., Nashville, TN.

Triple Trouble

Hardly a day goes by without higher statistics regarding the number of young people using drugs. Moreover, early use can bring on dependency and lead to addiction and death.

Many adolescents look at drugs as an instant remedy for a multitude of problems: home, school, or the world in which they live. Often drug use reflects a failure of relationships and lack of ability to shake peer pressure.

The "highs" and "lows" that drug use inflicts prohibit the user from living a normal life. People often take years of recovery to be freed from using drugs—just one more time.

Students have learned and re-learned about the effects of substance use and abuse; these range from mildly unpleasant to terrifying. At the onset of these fragile, early adolescent years we need to focus on the "why" some choose this experience and examine the consequences.

Supply students with experiences in which they listen to others and share their thinking. It's a time to reinforce every prevention skill available.

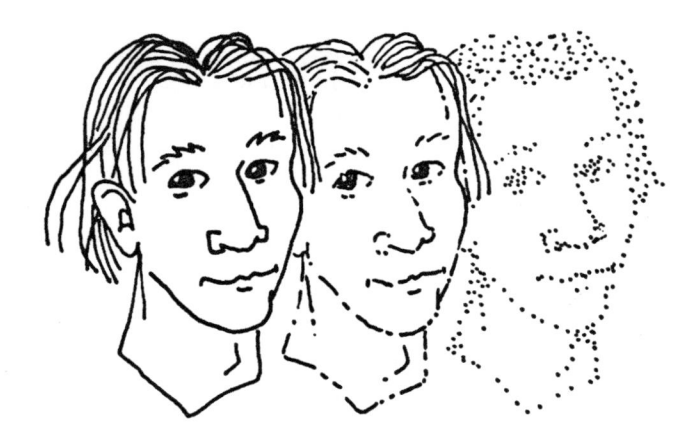

A Clear Message

SCENARIO

Shannon was a fun-loving twelve-year-old when she started smoking pot. She and her good friend Scott were experimenting. They thought marijuana was better than drinking alcohol because it was easier to hide.

Today, Shannon and Scott are no longer friends. He is in a rehabilitation (re-hab) program and takes night classes; she has moved to a "safer" town with her grandparents.

You've heard lots of horror stories similar to this. You might even know some of the people who use and abuse drugs.

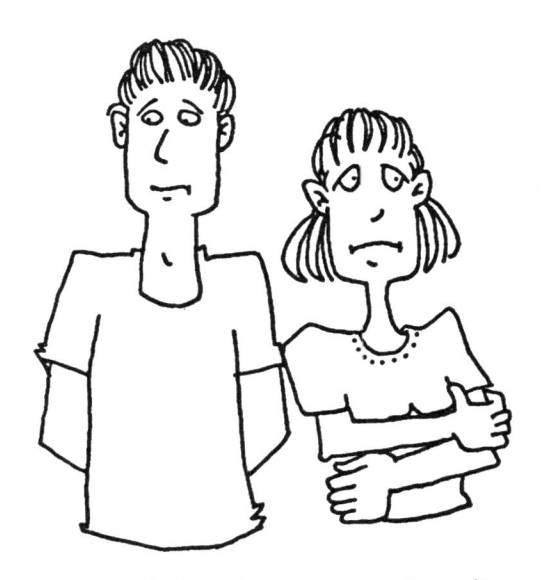

Shannon and Scott were addicted. Hopefully, while receiving help, they can get their lives back in order so they can once again be happy, healthy, and productive.

If you could have given a clear, "don't do it" message to them when they were eleven,

WHAT WOULD YOURS BE?

_____
_____
_____
_____
_____
_____

Focus Term: **Drug** — *A substance taken by mouth, injected, inhaled, or rubbed on the skin, that affects the way the mind or body normally works. It can alter your thinking or bodily functions.*

Focus Term: **Marijuana** — *A drug that comes from the flowering top and dried leaves of a cannabis, or hemp, plant.*

Serious Business

SCENARIO

Illegal drug use worsens many of society's problems. Drug users often lose interest in people and things that once had been very important to them. They become distant from friends and family. They lose interest in school. Hobbies and activities they once enjoyed are no longer fun.

Illegal drugs destroy the body. Drug users can become listless and overweight while using marijuana, or become stressed and suffer horrible sinus problems from using cocaine. Drug users can even overdose and die.

WHAT DO YOU KNOW?

Write a few paragraphs about the serious side of drug use.

_____
_____
_____
_____
_____
_____
_____
_____
_____
_____
_____
_____
_____

Focus Term: **Substance Abuse** — *The negative use, or overuse of drugs or alcohol.*

Thoughts on Why

SCENARIO

Somewhere between the ages of twelve and fifteen, countless young Americans have to decide whether or not to smoke marijuana. When we know so much about its bad effects, why would anyone want to?

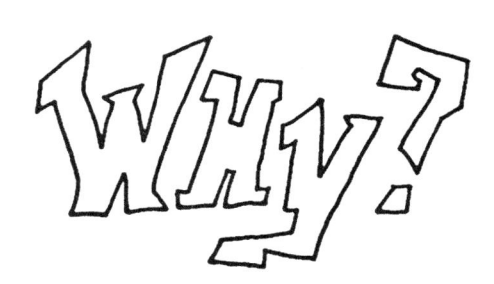

Kids smoke "pot"
- To respond to media and cultural pressures. "Do-Drugs" messages are found everywhere: magazines, pop songs, T-shirts, etc.
- To escape from problems of school or family
- To go along with the crowd; "everybody's doing it" kind of mentality; peer pressure
- To follow the example of a parent, older brother or sister, or other role model who has used drugs

WHAT DO YOU THINK?

Why do some young people use drugs?

1. _____

2. _____

3. _____

4. _____

Share some drug prevention thoughts with a classmate.

Health and Success

Joel's Story

SCENARIO

The coach told Joel, "You're pretty tough, but you'll have to beef up this year!"

The fifteen-year-old was the star quarterback on the JV team and hoped to be picked for varsity in the fall.

He began a vigorous training program and did all the right things: lifted weights, ran, got lots of sleep, and ate tons of healthy food. A month went by and the scales showed "no beef."

Some guys in the locker room told Joel what the pros do. It's weird, but worth a try, he thought. Joel was desperate.

It wasn't long before he found someone who could get him a supply. He took money out of savings and paid $200 for a drug called Anadrol. He got one month's supply of an anabolic steroid.

Now that's the beginning of Joel's story. HOW DO YOU THINK IT ENDS? If you don't know about steroids, do some research before writing a middle and ending for the story.

WRITE ABOUT IT

What happened to Joel was surprising . . .

_____
_____
_____
_____
_____
_____
_____
_____

Focus Term: **Anabolic Steroid** — *A drug used as a chemical boost for muscle development.*

Tips For Teens

More on drugs? "Oh no!" you say? Yes, when the topic is as life-threatening as drug use.

DID YOU KNOW?

About marijuana . . .

Marijuana is the most widely used illicit drug in the U.S. and tends to be the first illegal drug that teens use. It

- can impair or reduce memory and comprehension.
- can cause problems driving.
- can loosen you up so that you make a fool of yourself and do things you regret.
- has short-term effects including sleepiness, bloodshot eyes, and dry mouth
- has long-term effects including a risk of cancer and psychological dependence.
- can increase your appetite and make you gorge yourself on junk food, resulting in weight gain.
- blocks the messages going to your brain and alters your emotions, perceptions, vision, hearing, and coordination.

I learned, or relearned _____

_____

About inhalants . .

Inhalants are a diverse group of chemicals found in everyday consumer products. They are often a "gateway" to more addictive and dangerous drugs.

Short-term effects may include headache, nausea, muscle weakness, abdominal pain, and hallucinations.

Long-term use could result in hepatitis, violent behavior, suffocation, liver or kidney damage, and brain damage.

I learned, or relearned _____

_____

Focus Term: **Inhalant** — *A drug which is breathed in.*

Health and Success

More Tips For Teens

DID YOU KNOW?

About crack and cocaine . . .

Cocaine is a white powder that comes from the leaves of the South American coca plant. It belongs to a class of drugs called stimulants, which cause compulsive behavior.

Crack is a form of cocaine that has been chemically altered so it can be smoked. Both crack and cocaine are illegal substances.

Cocaine is snorted through the nasal passages or injected intravenously. Crack and cocaine are highly addictive and can dominate all aspects of life. The physical risks include heart attacks, strokes, respiratory failure, and brain seizures.

I learned, or relearned _____

_____

_____

_____

_____

About hallucinogens . . .

Hallucinogenic drugs are substances that distort reality for the user. A few of the better known are PCP, LSD, and peyote. The effects of these substances are unpredictable and often dangerous. Increased tolerance makes users of hallucinogens dangerous. Users must take more of a drug to get the same high, thereby making them more susceptible to overdose or to the side effects of the drugs. Convulsions, coma, or heart and lung failure are possible side effects.

I learned, or relearned _____

_____

_____

_____

_____

_____

Focus Term: **Addicted** — *Describes one who has a compulsive need for a habit-forming substance.*

A Dangerous Chew

SCENARIO

"I came to the ballpark, and I took the chewing tobacco out of my locker and put it in the trash can. I'm not going to touch the stuff. Life to me is more important than sticking tobacco in my mouth."

Cincinnati Reds' pitcher, Jeff Brantley

The U.S. Surgeon General and other medical experts have declared that smokeless tobacco has been linked to cancer of the mouth and throat. Thirty-eight-year-old Brett Butler is at least the eighth major league baseball player to develop cancer in recent years.

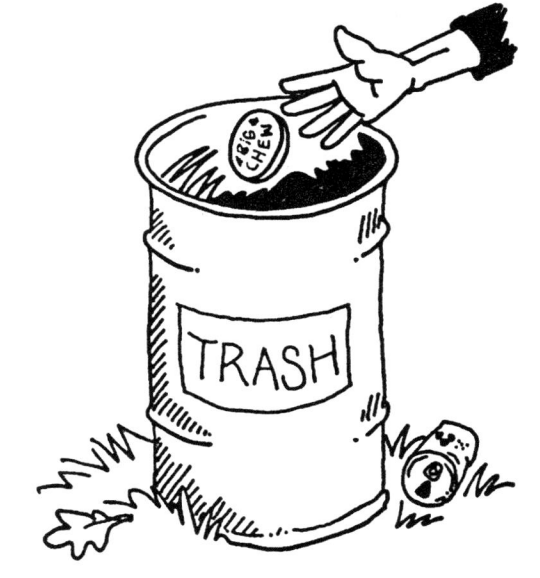

"Kids see athletes using the stuff," says Baseball Hall of Fame member Hank Aaron. "That can have a surprisingly devastating effect on young people."

THINK AND WRITE

Medical authorities cite studies showing a surprisingly high use of smokeless tobacco among both high school and elementary school students. What do you think about smokeless tobacco? _____

___

___

___

___

___

___

___

___

Focus Term: **Smokeless Tobacco** — *A form of tobacco that is not meant to be smoked; it is held in the mouth or chewed like gum*

Chewed Out

SCENARIO

"This product may cause gum disease and tooth loss"
(Warning found on chewing tobacco containers)

His face is scarred by six cancer operations. He has no teeth and can't taste. The sixty-six-year-old man has trouble talking and hearing. Bill Tuttle, a gifted former major league baseball player, played eleven seasons for Detroit, Kansas City, and Minnesota. He blames all of his troubles on "spit tobacco."

For years Bill chewed non-stop. It was part of playing the game—like hot dogs and peanuts. "It was always a dirty habit," says Bill, "but now it's deadly."

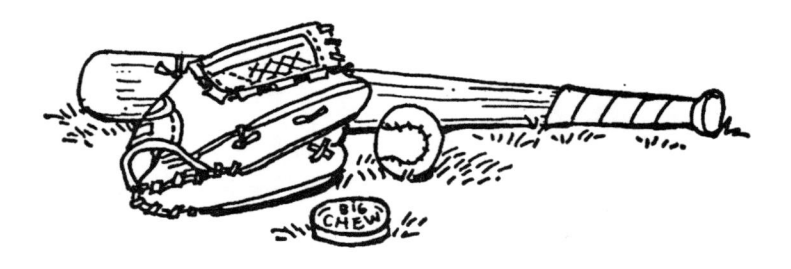

A large poster in the Pittsburgh Pirates Clubhouse shows Bill Tuttle "then" and "now"—the glory and the gory. The picture is worth a thousand words, claim players who have kicked the habit.

LET'S IMAGINE

You are a Little League coach and work with little kids every day. These young, impressionable boys and girls love baseball and watch the major league games on TV. Give them your message about smokeless tobacco. Get more information if you don't know the facts!

"Hey kids, listen up! . . ."

Focus Term: **Warning** — *To give notice to a person of impending evil or danger.*

Smoke Rises/Numbers Increase

SCENARIO

The facts are grisly!

- Heart Disease
- Lung, Larynx, Esophageal, Pancreatic, and Kidney Cancer
- Emphysema
- Chronic Bronchitis
- Everyday yucky stuff: bad breath, dirty stains on teeth and fingers, burns, expense
- Addiction

The scenario reads like a Steven King thriller. Even Joe Camel says "kids shouldn't smoke."

Although the anti-smoking movement is on a roll, the statistics are not good. The number of teen smokers is rising. The nonsmoking public wonders:

WRITE ABOUT IT

Why are people smoking when they know the consequences? What are the temptations?

_____
_____
_____
_____
_____

What can be done to curb cigarette purchases made by adolescents?

_____
_____
_____
_____
_____

Focus Term: **Temptation** — *Something that entices or allures.*

Health and Success

Bad And Sad

SCENARIO

Robyn and Liz were on their way to the convenience store on the corner. They were planning to ask an older kid to buy cigarettes for them.

While they waited for someone to come along, a ragged, dirty old man slowly walked by. He stopped at a trash can and started going through the garbage. The girls noticed that he put a few things in his pockets, then something in his mouth. He lit the tiny butt of a cigarette, puffed on it and slowly started to amble away.

"Did you see that?" whispered Liz as she watched in amazement.

"Yuck!" I knew smoking was an addiction, but that was the pits," said Robyn. "Maybe we ought to think twice about this."

"It's bad and it's sad," agreed her friend.

The old man stopped and turned toward them. "I see you watchin' me, girls. Let me tell you somethin' about these poison sticks."

HOW DOES IT END?

Finish the story. What did the old man tell Robyn and Liz about cigarette smoking?

"It all started when . . .

_____
_____
_____
_____
_____
_____
_____

Focus Term: **Underage** — *Lacking the required age of legal maturity.*

About Alcohol

QUICK FACTS

On the lines below, add a personal reaction. Tell what you know about each statement.

1. **Know the laws**—If you are under twenty-one years old, it is illegal to buy or possess alcohol. _____
_____
_____

2. **Get the straight facts**—A twelve ounce can of beer has as much alcohol as a glass of wine, a shot of whiskey or a wine cooler.
_____
_____
_____

3. **Know the risks**—Alcoholism is a disease. It blocks the messages to the brain and can damage your liver. Alcoholism can cause you personal and school problems. _____
_____
_____

4. **Play it safe**—Drinking can lead to intoxication and increase the risk of serious injury. Never drive with someone who has had even one drink. _____
_____
_____

5. **Be a friend**—If you think someone you know has a drinking problem, help him or her get help. Urge your friend to talk to an adult or school counselor. _____
_____
_____

6. **Be aware**—Know that alcohol does not provide the adventure and glamour as is often portrayed. _____
_____
_____

Focus Term: **Alcoholism** — *A diseased condition resulting from the excessive use of and dependence on alcoholic beverages.*

The Confrontation

SCENARIO

"You do it, so why shouldn't I?" shouted the fourteen-year-old. "You're a hypocrite."

Matt's dad caught him sneaking into the house long after the curfew on which they had agreed. Matt and some friends had had a few beers down at the pond and things had gotten rough and silly. Matt had fallen in the water; he looked like a mess.

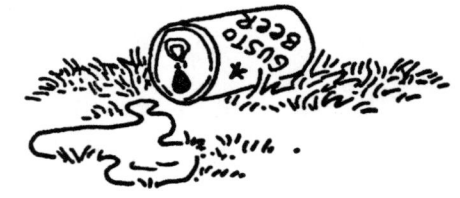

Parents are usually clear about not wanting their children to use drugs, but sometimes it's harder to be tough about alcohol. It is a legal substance for adults, and many parents drink it. Alcohol is also an important part of many religious observances and family gatherings.

Although we may view alcohol as a substance less dangerous than drugs, alcohol-related accidents are one of the leading causes of death among young people.

TO WRITE ABOUT

How can Matt and his dad resolve their anger with each other? Be specific and be reasonable.

_____
_____
_____
_____
_____
_____
_____
_____
_____
_____

Hey! Put That Out!

SCENARIO

Mr. Ross was a well-liked school custodian for many years. He was a heavy smoker and could often be found working in his smoke-filled shop.

Last week, Mr. Ross died of lung cancer. Yesterday his wife died of a stroke. The doctor said Mrs. Ross, a non-smoker, had serious lung damage and also suffered from atherosclerosis.

Smoking is a killer habit that can kill you, whether you smoke or not. It is like a serial killer running loose.

We are all aware of the long-term risks to which smokers expose themselves, but smoking hurts everyone around them as well. Studies have shown a direct link between second-hand smoke and other diseases such as atherosclerosis. Findings indicate the arteries of people exposed to passive smoke thicken at a faster rate than those of people not exposed.

Passive smokers may account for more than 53,000 deaths annually. This is tragic for innocent bystanders—especially young and unborn children.

TAKE ACTION!

Write an article for your school newspaper or news flash for a school radio program about "second-hand smoke." Make it tough; tell all you know!

_____
_____
_____
_____
_____
_____

Focus Word: **Passive Smokers** — *Those people who do not actually smoke cigarettes, but breathe in the smoke of others.*

Think Tank

SCENARIO

Discuss this in a group of three or four.

Do you have any bad habits—things you know you shouldn't do but you can't seem to stop doing? Maybe you bite your nails or eat too many sweets. Have you ever tried to break a bad habit? How did that feel? Were you successful? How did you do?

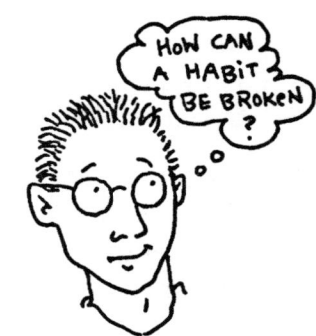

For most people, habits are not easy to break. How much more difficult do you think it is to break a habit like smoking, or drinking alcohol? Smoking and drinking are not just habits. Cigarettes contain nicotine, a highly addictive drug. Alcohol is also addictive. Even when smokers and alcoholics want to quit, their bodies still crave the drugs.

Cigarettes, drugs, and alcohol are habit forming. Do users know it is unhealthy before they begin?

_____

_____

When a person forms a dangerous habit, how hard is it to break it?

_____

_____

HOW CAN A HABIT BE BROKEN?

_____

_____

_____

_____

_____

_____

_____

Focus Word: **Habit** — *A tendency to act in a certain way; repetition of an act.*

CHAPTER THREE

Help!

38	**TEACHER'S PAGE**
39	*Our Violent World* — How can you reduce violence? Think and write.
40	*The Never-Never List* — How can you stay safe? Think and write.
41	*Dear Denzel* — Get involved! Write a letter!
42	*More than Watching TV* — Liz's scenario . . . Baby-sitting, that is!
43	*Doggone Shot* — Gun Safety . . . Think and write.
44	*The Probe* — Racial problems . . . Any ideas?
45	*In Self-Defense* — Physical violence . . . Think and share.
46	*Been There* — Have you? How do you protect yourself?
47	*When Enough is Enough* — Verbal abuse . . . Write and go from there.
48	*Poetic Justice* — Personal translation . . . Can you relate?

Help!

"The richest, longest-lived, best-protected, most resourceful civilization, with the highest degree of insight into its own technology, is on its way to becoming the most frightened. Has there ever been, one wonders, a society that produced more uncertainty more often about everyday life?"

—Aaron Wildavsky on risk in the American culture

There was an era when families concerned with city crime and violence moved to the suburbs. Today, violence once found only in metropolitan areas has also moved into the suburbs—and even beyond, into the countryside.

Injury and violence are currently a leading cause of death for teenagers. How can they learn to protect themselves?

The following ten pages provide subject matter of a serious nature. They require students to think, then react to various scenarios that focus on impending dangers.

To protect vulnerable students, follow-up discussions should be de-personalized. However, some instances may require that a school nurse or social worker be alerted.

The mental health of middle school age children is fragile. Don't hesitate to offer help, guidance, and reassurance, but leave counseling and intervention for the appropriate professionals.

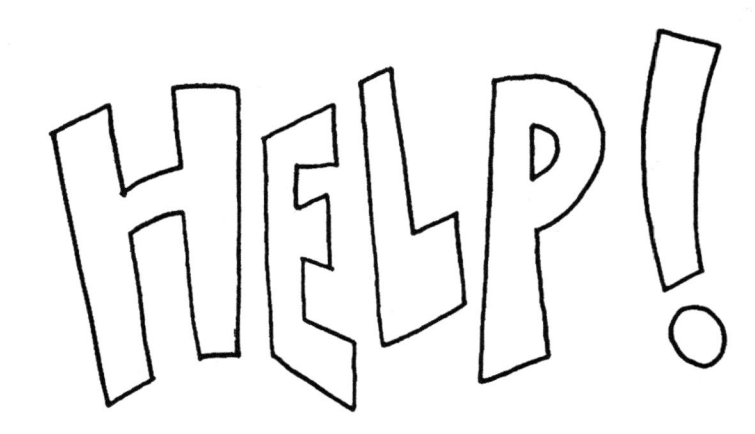

Our Violent World

SCENARIO

A physician was recently asked what new diseases pose a threat to young people. His reply was surprising: "The largest epidemic we have on our hands now is violence."

Statistics tell us that injury and violence are the leading causes of death for adolescents. These young victims die of accidents, suicide, or homicide. In some areas of the country, the streets, the schools, and even some houses are not safe.

THINK AND WRITE

Choose one of the following topics to write about.

Things We Can Do To:
- Use words, not force
- Get out of an abusive relationship
- Learn to handle anger
- Decrease violence on TV
- Not be afraid to seek help when needed

Your Space

_____
_____
_____
_____
_____
_____
_____
_____

Focus Word: **Victim** — A *sufferer from any injurious or adverse action.*

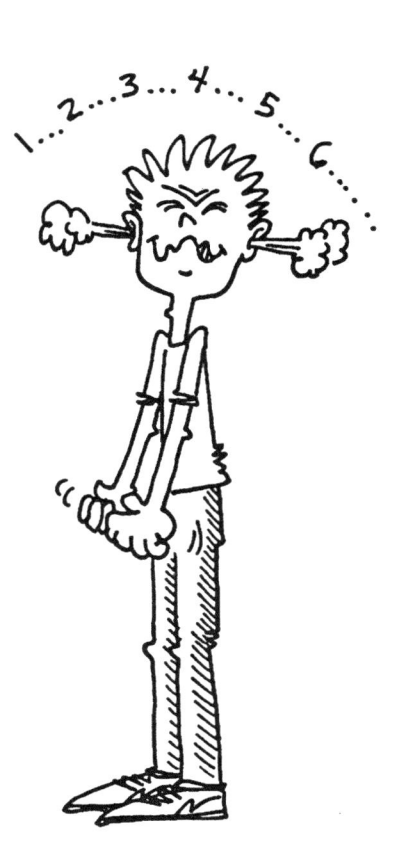

Health and Success

The Never-Never List

SCENARIO

Remember back when you were a little kid and the "never-never" list was recited to you whenever you went anywhere?

Never talk to strangers.

Never accept rides from strangers.

Never take candy from strangers.

The list went on and on. Now, even though you're older, the world is tougher. The violence we hear and read about in the media—or see in our own communities—is threatening our own sense of security.

THINK AND WRITE

The "never-never" list is growing. Add things about which to be careful—things to watch out for in the neighborhood.

1. Never walk in unlit areas at night.
2. Never flash money.
3. Never travel alone in dangerous areas.
4. _____
5. _____
6. _____
7. _____
8. _____
9. _____
10. _____

Review your list with that of a classmate. Are they similar?

Focus Word: **Security**— *Freedom from danger or risk.*

Dear Denzel

SCENARIO

"Much has been reported about the escalating rate of youth crime and violence, with such terms as 'super predators' and 'kids without a conscience' used to describe America's troubled teen-age population," says Denzel Washington.

This well-known actor believes that providing at-risk youth with a program of organized, supervised activities is the first step towards reaching out to help.

As a member of the Board of Governors of Boys and Girls Clubs of America, he tells of nine hundred new locations, bringing the total to more than eighteen hundred. Most Clubs are in urban and inner-city neighborhoods where kids are at greatest risk. Young people are taught how to resist peer pressure and avoid violence.

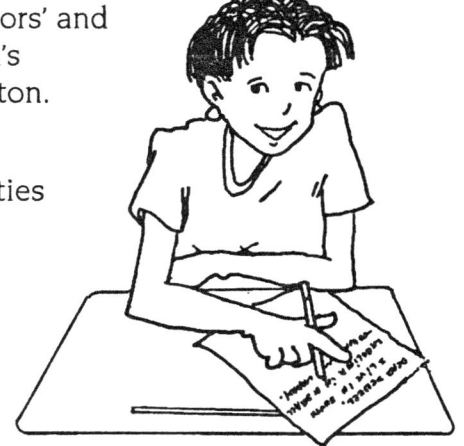

The actor is himself a former Club member and knows the positive influence Boys and Girls Clubs have on kids. Thanks to efforts such as his, more than 2.4 million kids benefit from an investment in a safer future.

TO DO

On the back of this sheet, write a letter to Denzel Washington, in care of (c/o) a Boys and Girls Club in your city.

Choose one of the following to tell him:
1. About the Boys and Girls Club in your city
2. About the problems in your community and why you need such a club
3. What you think of his message

Focus Word: **At Risk Youth** — *Young people who, because of their age or circumstances are in potential danger.*

More Than Watching TV

—Baby-sitting that is!

SCENARIO

Liz answered the Addison's phone, but she heard no voice at the other end. She heard only the sounds of heavy breathing and moaning. She hung up and told the children, "If the phone rings again, don't answer it. I'll get it."

A few minutes later it happened again. What should she do?

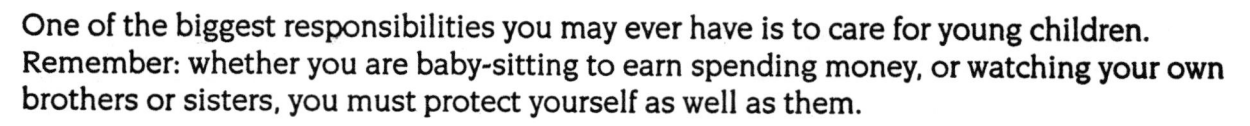

One of the biggest responsibilities you may ever have is to care for young children. Remember: whether you are baby-sitting to earn spending money, or watching your own brothers or sisters, you must protect yourself as well as them.

Baby-sitting is more than watching TV!

Some On The Job Tips:

1. When accepting a new job, check out the family. Are they known to anyone you know? Have you agreed upon how you will be paid?
2. Clarify transportation arrangements and have a back-up in case the parents appear to have been drinking.
3. Keep doors locked; never let in strangers.
4. Don't invite friends to visit; this is a job.
5. Get phone numbers where the parents can be reached.
6. Have other emergency numbers on hand—especially a close neighbor.
7. Familiarize yourself with the layout of the house.
8. Don't hesitate to call police if you hear suspicious noises.
9. Get the kids and yourself out fast if you smell smoke. Call "911" from a neighbor's home.
10. Always give your family the phone number and let them know when you expect to be home.
11. Report all unusual occurrences to the parents when they return.

HOW YOU DID IT

Tell about a difficult baby-sitting experience you once had.
How did you handle your responsibility?

Focus Word: **Responsibility** — *A burden of obligation; answerable or accountable for a situation.*

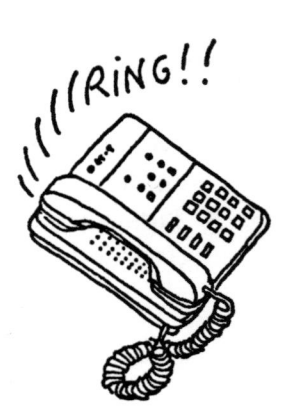

Doggone Shot

SCENARIO

Dateline Martin County, KY—Philip Smith is recuperating from a hunting accident in which his friend's dog set off a shotgun, hitting Smith in both legs. Rusty, a fifteen month old spaniel, stepped on the trigger as he and his owner, John Phillips, tussled over a felled bird.

This news brief is a good example of how dangerous guns can be, even in what began as a nonviolent situation.

Hardly a day goes by that we don't read about accidents or fatalities that result from the use or misuse of firearms. The victims are of all ages. Many innocent bystanders are killed by being at the wrong place at the wrong time.

Crimes of passion, domestic violence, gang wars—the list goes on and on. You also hear stories of accidents such as Rusty the dog "shooting" the gun.

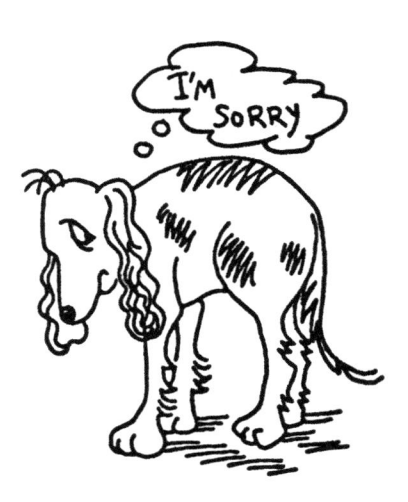

THINKING SPACE

Statistics tell us that fifty one percent of gun owners keep their guns loaded. Firearms at home are forty-three times more likely to kill friends or family than to be used in self defense. What do you think about gun safety and gun control? Is it a problem where you live? How can you stay safe?

WRITING SPACE

_____
_____
_____
_____
_____
_____
_____

Focus Word: **Fire Arm** — A gun from which a projectile is fired; small arms.

The Probe

SCENARIO

Dateline Waterbury, CT—Racial and ethnic slurs have been spray-painted on a wall at the West Side Middle School twice in one week, officials say. The graffiti has been removed; a probe is under way.

It is a grim reality that hate crimes and misdemeanors occur far too frequently in our society. The Waterbury incident was disturbing and stressful to the students' mental health and an outrage to parents and faculty. Ethnic and minority groups viewed the graffiti with revulsion.

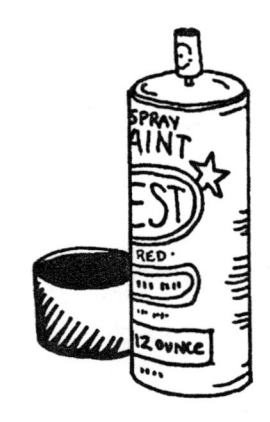

What is the source of this anger? How can that school eliminate hate?

YOUR IDEAS

Some causes of anger and hostility are:

1. _____
2. _____
3. _____
4. _____
5. _____

How can schools work towards a positive influence?

1. _____
2. _____
3. _____
4 _____
5. _____

Focus Word: **Misdemeanor** — *Misbehavior; a misdeed; a serious offense, but less serious than a felony.*

In Self-Defense

SCENARIO

An instant before the final buzzer, Andy made one last shot to win the game ninety-six to ninety-five. The gym erupted with excited fans pouring onto the court.

An angry, hostile crowd from the opposing side started pushing cheerleaders and yelling obscenities at the winning team.

Things got tough; tempers flared and fists flew. Andy and his teammates got into the action and threw a few punches. Suddenly Andy felt a sharp pain in his chest. Blood spurted from a knife hole in the middle of his number—32!

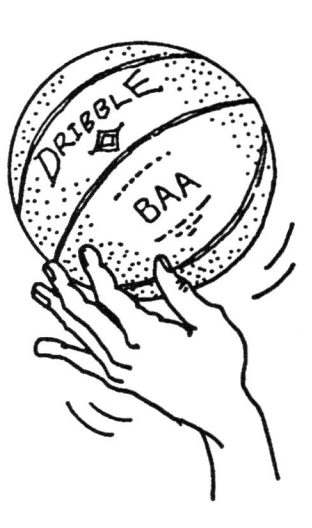

THINK ABOUT

Andy was lucky; he recovered. Both schools went through a period of counseling on violence and focused on the outrage students were feeling.

Did you ever feel you needed to "get tough" in self-defense? How did it work out? What else could you have done?

SHARE WHAT HAPPENED

_____
_____
_____
_____
_____
_____
_____

Focus Word: **Counseling** — *Opinion or instruction given in directing the judgement or conduct of another.*

Health and Success

Been There! Have You?

SCENARIO

A seventh grader wrote to "Dear Sally" explaining how his school was full of weapons and drugs. "Scared" asked for advice on how to protect himself.

The advice was as follows: (If you or someone you know has "been there," tell how it was handled.)

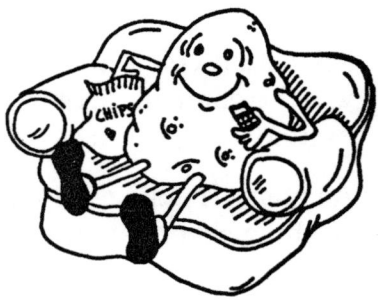

1. If you don't know karate, and you are a couch potato, take a course in self-defense. Make sure you don't come across as a push-over! Been there? _____

2. If you are approached about drugs, don't make eye contact. Shake your head "no" and keep on walking. Be calm and matter of fact. Politeness is not important in this situation! Been there? _____

3. If there's a fight—get out of there! Someone may have a weapon. Cool kids might hang around to watch. Smart kids get out of town . . . fast! You can tell an adult, but don't offer your name. Been there? _____

4. If you are ever backed into a corner, scream your head off! It will draw attention and you are less likely to be a victim. After you warn bystanders, practice a really loud scream! Been there? _____

5. Never be afraid to ask for advice or to tell an adult about a dangerous situation. You know the cool ones you can trust. Been there? _____

6. Be alert! Don't go into stairwells or restrooms alone. If you are not with a friend and feel threatened, walk behind a group for protection. Been there? _____

Focus Word: **Couch Potato** — *A slang expression for one who lies around snacking and watching TV; someone who is usually not physically fit.*

When Enough Is Enough

SCENARIO

"Get out of my sight!"

"I hate you!"

"You drive me nuts!"

"You're so stupid!"

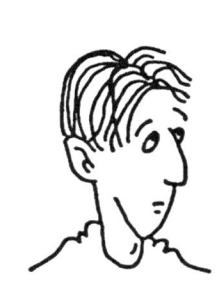

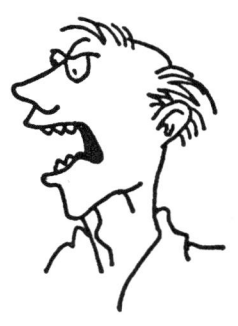

Comments such as these can make people feel unloved and worthless. Parents who express these kinds of negative words to their children are often blaming them for problems in their own lives.

Physical abuse could be the next step. Severe punishments and beatings can cause serious injury. Some parents can't handle the responsibilities of raising children, because they have too many other problems in their own lives. Some just expect too much from their children.

Dysfunction in the family can be caused by a number of things. Problems such as alcohol, drug abuse, poverty, divorce, gambling, death, and mental illness can be responsible. Sometimes it's just how parents were raised themselves.

It's important for young people to know to ask for help. Sure, it may be embarrassing—something you don't want the other kids to know about—but a trustworthy person can help.

WHAT TO DO

But if you feel frightened and confused, talk to an adult you can trust. Explain what is happening in your life. At some point in our lives we all need help; yours may be now. Start by writing here.

I wish _____

_____

_____

_____

_____

Focus Word: **Dysfunctional Family** — *A family in which members are not behaving in an appropriate manner. Children often have to change their behavior to cope with problems.*

Poetic Justice

Fourteen-year-old Jamie won the local newspaper's anti-violence contest with this powerful poem.

Love, Violence and Us

The wind can be violent
At the height of a storm.
The breeze can be soft,
caressing and warm.

The wave can be playful
on a bright summer's day;
Then crashes with violence,
Breaking ships in its way.

The flakes are pure magic
In the light falling snow.
An avalanche chases
The skiers below.

The boy with his visions
Takes time for a flower;
Becoming a terrorist
Intense with his power.

An explosion of force;
A contrast so great.
Can this be what happens
When love turns to hate?

We know we can't name it–
The violence in weather.
But maybe through love
We can tame "us" forever.

GET THINKING

Give some thought to Jamie's poem and translate the ideas into what is happening in your community. Write a poem about what you read, see, or feel is happening where you live.

_____
_____
_____

MORE

How can we "tame" violence?_____
_____
_____

Focus Word: **Violence** — Rough or injurious action or treatment.

CHAPTER FOUR

Big Changes—Big Choices

50	**TEACHER'S PAGE**
51	*What's On Your Mind?* Any questions? Get some answers!
52	*Girl Talk* Growing up... In your own words.
53	*Guy Talk* Growing up... In your own words.
54	*Three Girls* Which one are you? How do the others feel?
55	*Just For Guys* Growing pains... What advice can you give?
56	*The Crush* Creative story ending... You decide!
57	*Don't Be Ignorant* Here are the facts... Consider yourself informed!
58	*The Teen Dilemmas* What's your worry? Stop and prioritize.
59	*Teen Moms* Katherine's scenario... Write back.
60	*"How Am I Doing?"* Check Sheet on Decision Making... How can you improve?

Big Changes—Big Choices

"Kids in danger—Handle with care."

Teachers and parents don't need a road sign such as this to remind them of adolescents in peril.

Adolescents are exposed to a lot of "trash" from which to pick and choose. They need to learn the facts and be taught how to weigh the consequences.

Scientific information and health facts must come from the school curriculum. The following pages provide provocative, health-related subject matter to enrich the minds of young adolescents. These materials may be passed along to a health teacher for implementation. Lots of heavy discussion may evolve if used in separate male/female groups.

The author Robie Harris reminds us that "hiding reality might depict sex as wrong, shameful, secret, or dirty."

Parents should be the first and foremost educators for human sexuality. Unfortunately, that does not always happen. Some feel inadequate or embarrassed; others may refer back to the stork or "birds and bees."

The streets, the media, or peer groups then take over. The fears, jokes, and questions from adolescents need addressing before it's too late. Young people are often ignorant of the facts that affect the rest of their lives.

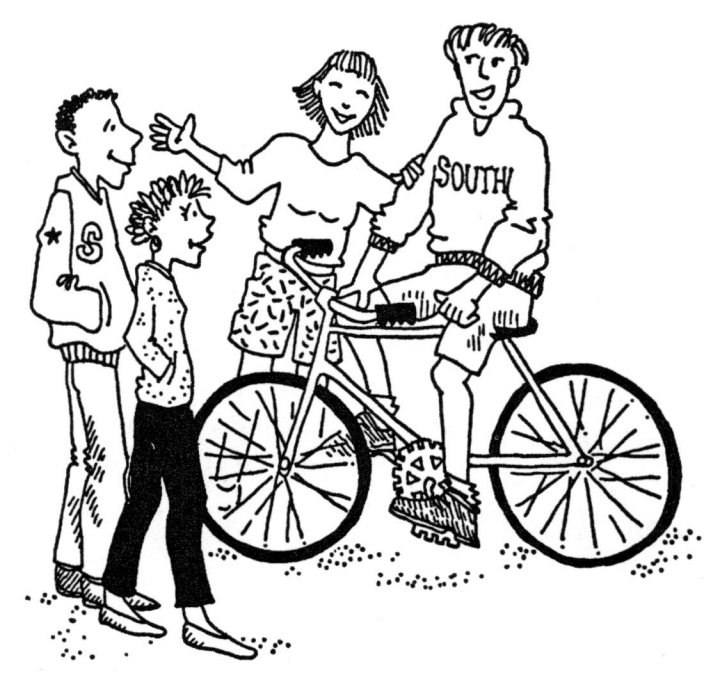

What's On Your Mind

SCENARIO

What do you and your friends mostly talk about when you are hanging out? Clothes? Baseball? School? Parents? Weather? The opposite sex?

During the next few years your life will change in many ways. You will slowly (sometimes quickly!) develop new ideas, new friends, and a new body. There are exciting changes taking place in your life. Both girls and boys will find they are interested in sexual subjects.

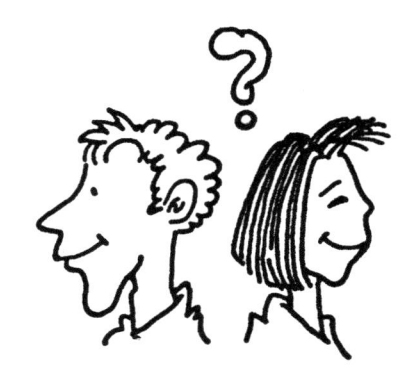

Be sure that you understand what's happening; lack of information can result in your doing some things you really don't mean to do.

WRITE ABOUT IT

What's on your mind? Some things you would like to know more about:

1. _____

2. _____

3. _____

4. _____

5. _____

Share your questions with your health teacher, parent or an adult you can trust. Or, why not go to the library alone or with a special friend; take out a book that will help you clear up what's on your mind.

Focus Word: **Sexuality** — *The recognition or emphasizing of sexual matters.*

Health and Success

©1999 by Incentive Publications, Inc., Nashville, TN.

Girl Talk

SCENARIO

Somewhere between the ages of nine and sixteen your body—inside and outside—makes some big changes. This process is called puberty. Different glands start producing hormones. These chemicals are sent through your blood stream to many parts of your body; they influence the way your body develops and the emotions you feel.

A more adult figure will emerge.

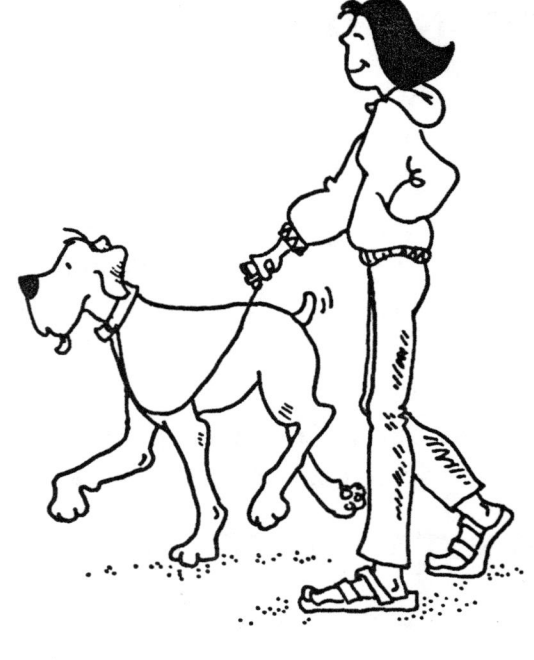

IN YOUR OWN WORDS

The part of growing up I like is

_____
_____
_____
_____
_____
_____

The part of growing up I don't like is

_____
_____
_____
_____
_____
_____
_____
_____

Focus Word: **Puberty** — *The time in which sexual maturity occurs.*

Guy Talk

SCENARIO

You have reached the age of puberty; the time when your body becomes more like that of a man. Our bodies are always changing, but never more than between the ages of ten and seventeen. This time of transition can be very traumatic.

It's a time when you grow taller and your voice changes. As your voice box expands the sounds you make may squeak and crackle as they get deeper.

Hair begins to grow on your body in places that have always been smooth; you think about shaving.

IN YOUR OWN WORDS

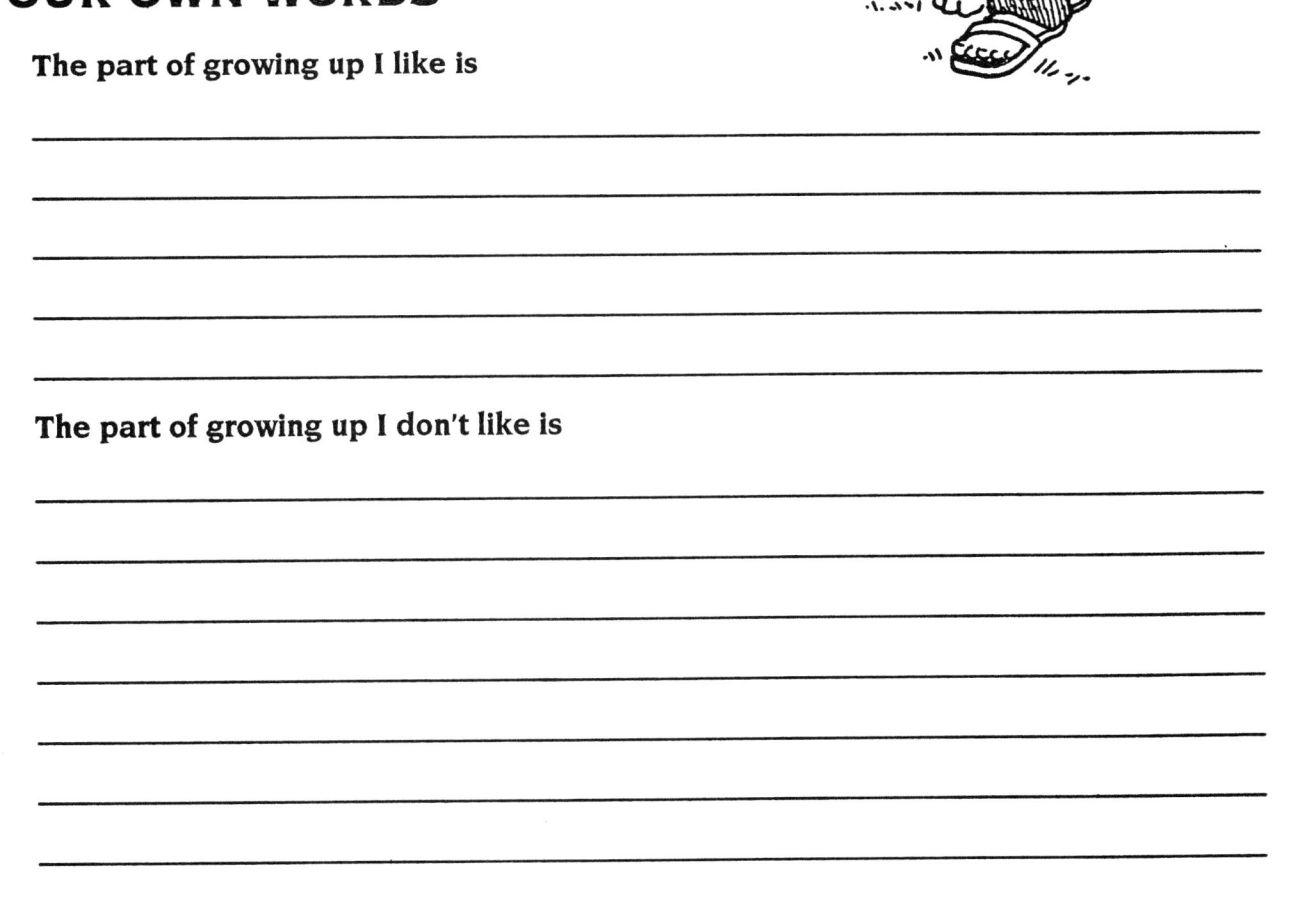

The part of growing up I like is

_____
_____
_____
_____
_____

The part of growing up I don't like is

_____
_____
_____
_____
_____
_____
_____

Focus Word: **Transition** — *A passage from one state or form to another.*

Three Girls

SCENARIO

The following girls are sitting in a health class.

Kid # 1–Kelly is twelve years old and has not yet developed. She is looking to her left, then to her right. She is wondering, "When's that going to happen to me?"

_____
_____
_____
_____

Kid # 2–Trish, who is developing, is looking to her left, then to her right. She is wondering "What in the heck is happening to me?" She feels conspicuous.

_____
_____
_____
_____

Kid # 3–Cheryl is not looking around at her classmates; she is listening to the health teacher. She knows about and is comfortable with what is going on with her body.

_____
_____
_____

Confusion is common at this stage of development. "Normal" doesn't seem to exist. Some of your friends may have a bodies like movie stars, while others haven't developed at all.

Some feel embarrassed by the changes taking place; others think it's great.

Where are you? Are you Kid # 1, Kid #2 or Kid # 3? Sexuality affects us differently at different ages. How do you think the girls feel? Give each of them a few words of reassurance.

Focus Word: **Developed** — *To grow or expand to a more advanced level.*

Just For Guys

SCENARIO

For years Adam, Aaron and Andy have called themselves the "Three Aces." As neighbors they did everything together; climbed trees, caught frogs, camped out and built a fort not to be equaled.

The "Three Aces," now in middle school, still hang out together when not busy with other things. There are some big changes though:

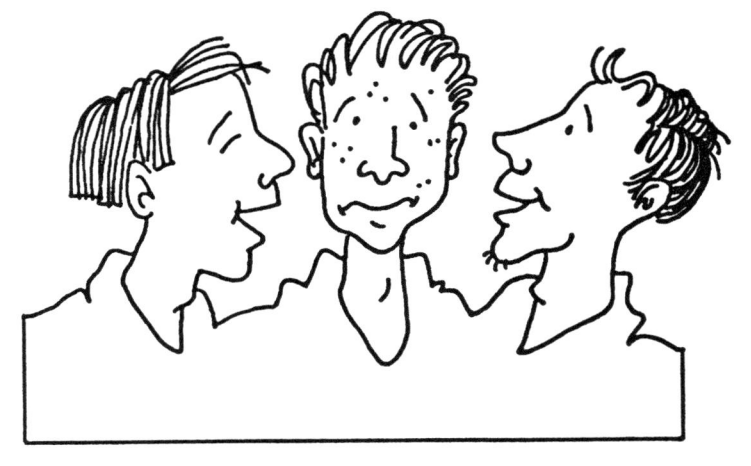

Adam has a deep voice and is hoping to shave soon. The guys tease him about the "peach fuzz," but he feels proud.

_____

_____

_____

Aaron talks about "chicks" a lot. He likes kissing and all the stuff that goes along with it. He brags a lot these days.

_____

_____

_____

Andy feels left out. He keeps looking for hair and muscles and girls, but is ashamed none of the three are appearing in his life. He sweats a lot these days and has acne.

_____

_____

_____

The "Three Aces" notice that growing up seems to happen later for boys than it does for girls. Some guys worry about things that have or have not happened to them. Can you give some advice to these three guys?

Focus Word: **Acne** — *A skin condition, involving pimples and blackheads, which occurs when pores are blocked.*

The Crush

SCENARIO

Cheryl had a crush on Brian. He didn't pay much attention to her, but that was OK. She stared dreamily at the back of his head every day in math class.

One day Brian followed Cheryl out of the room and pleasantly surprised her by asking if they could do homework together that afternoon.

"Why don't we go up to your house," he suggested.

Cheryl agreed—reluctantly. She knew her Mom was at work and would not like the idea. The rule was no kids in the condo when no adults were there.

She spread her books out on the kitchen table, then brought out cokes and snacks.

"Why don't we go into your bedroom where it's comfortable?" proposed Brian.

"No way, that's not possible!"

"Come on. Then the homework won't be so boring," he argued.

Cheryl thought for a moment. Maybe he won't like me or ever want to be with me again if I don't. But then . . .

WHAT DO YOU THINK?

You finish the story. Write the dialogue for Cheryl and Brian.

_____

_____

_____

_____

More: Why did you finish the story the way you did? _____

_____

_____

Focus Word: **Crush** — *Strong feelings about a member of the opposite sex.*

Don't Be Ignorant

SCENARIO

AIDS. It's one of the most serious diseases known to our society. There is no known cure.

AIDS (Acquired Immune Deficiency Syndrome) is caused by the human immunodeficiency virus (HIV). People die of pneumonia and various forms of cancer because of the damage done to their body's immune system.

A frightening statistic: more than thirty percent of those with AIDS are in their late teens and early twenties.

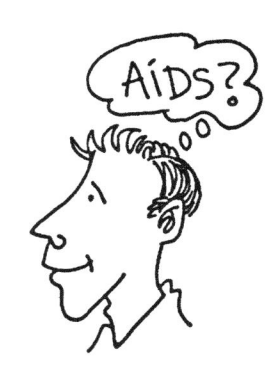

WHAT DO YOU KNOW?

Mark the following "true" or "false."
As far as it is known:

_____ Three possible ways to get AIDS are sex, tainted blood transfusions, and shared needles among drug users.

_____ People who have AIDS don't always know they have it.

_____ The virus that causes AIDS was first discovered as recently as 1981.

_____ Kissing will not give you HIV.

_____ Many people who have AIDS are treated badly by society.

_____ Some new medications are keeping people with AIDS alive longer.

_____ Newborn babies can get HIV from their mothers.

_____ People with AIDS need our compassion.

Answers to Quiz: If you answered "true" to all statements, you are 100% correct. You know the facts about AIDS and HIV.

Now go back and place an asterisk (*) beside one of the statements. Discuss your thoughts about that topic in the space below.

I think/believe/wonder/hope . . . _____

_____

_____

Focus Word: **AIDS** — *Acquired Immune Deficiency Syndrome.*
Focus Word: **HIV** — *Human Immunodeficiency Virus.*

The Teen Dilemmas

SCENARIO

At some point during the teenage years boys and girls go through lots of natural—sometimes embarrassing—changes.

Both sexes start cranking up hormone production; that can give you lots to think about!

A current poll of young people listed the following as dilemmas. Read the list, then number them ranking #1 as most important in your life to #13 as least important.

SHOULD YOU:

_____ worry about which jeans are cool?

_____ ask (someone) to go out?

_____ drink beer at a party?

_____ make out with (someone) at a party?

_____ read teen age magazines for advice?

_____ be more concerned with health issues?

_____ take a stand on second-hand smoke?

_____ think more seriously about the consequences of what you do?

_____ think about having sex as an awesome issue?

_____ worry less about what others in your group think?

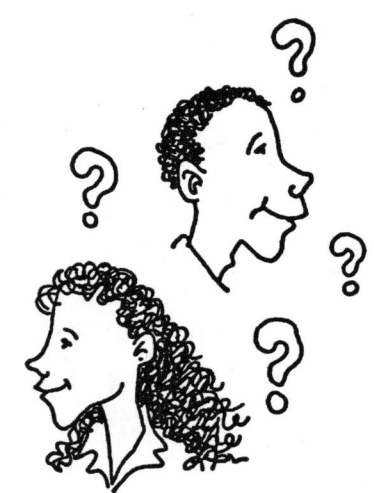

_____ be your own person?

_____ stand firm on your morals and values?

NOW—GO BACK AND DECIDE:

Number 1 is most important because _____
_____

Number 13 is least important because _____
_____

Focus Word: **Dilemma** — *A situation requiring a choice between equally desirable or undesirable alternatives.*

Teen Moms

SCENARIO

Katherine had dated John for about two weeks when they decided to sleep together. She was uncomfortable about her decision, and her life became more difficult when she found that she was pregnant.

When she told him, they had an argument and he has not called since then. It has been a week and she is feeling desperate.

Katherine is only fifteen. How does she tell her parents? What can she do?

It's too late to remind Katherine that when she chose to be sexually active she should have considered the consequences.

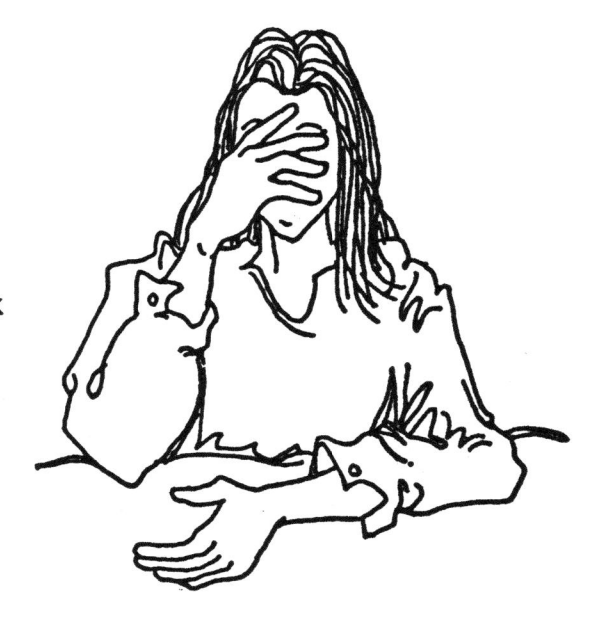

WRITE ABOUT IT

_____
_____
_____
_____
_____
_____
_____
_____
_____
_____
_____
_____
_____
_____

"How Am I Doing?" Check Sheet

SCENARIO

Lots of teens do an O.K. job in the decision-making department. Some could do better. Where are you?

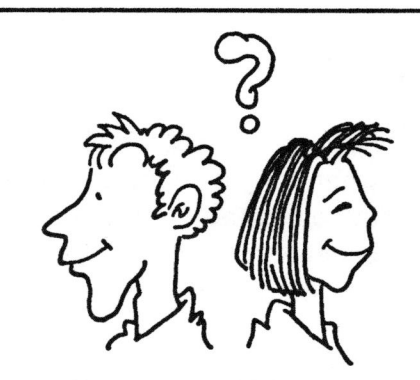

WHAT DO YOU THINK?

	Yes	Sometimes	No
1. I like hanging out in groups.			
2. I like casual dating.			
3. I'd like to go out.			
4. I'd feel tied down by a serious relationship.			
5. I never feel out of control.			
6. I feel comfortable saying "no!"			
7. I enjoy lots of things besides dating.			
8. I think life at this time is O.K. without a boy or girlfriend.			

Well, how are you doing? (Your privacy will be respected)

I feel that _____

_____

_____

I need to _____

_____

_____

I learned _____

_____

_____

CHAPTER FIVE

The Need To Know

62	**TEACHER'S PAGE**
63	*Hotline Available* — Facing a crisis? Share with a friend.
64	*Nikki's Story* — Support organizations... What do you think?
65	*Plan To Be Happy* — What can you do to be happy? Break it down.
66	*Hassle Log* — How can you control your anger? Analyze your actions!
67	*The Suicide* — Judy's scenario... Symptoms and solutions.
68	*Be Someone Who Cares* — Suicide... Signs to alert you.
69	*No Bikini For Paula* — Eating disorders... List some trigger thoughts.
70	*Getting Help* — Answers to... How, who, where?
71	*Rate Your Life* — From where you stand. Think and write.
72	*The Negative Chain* — If... then Can you see the consequences?

Health and Success

©1999 by Incentive Publications, Inc., Nashville, TN.

The Need To Know

Youth is not carefree these days; the problems are more hazardous than those in the past. Some kids have family support and understanding. Others learn early "on the street."

Suicide is the third most common form of death among young people. It's final, and it doesn't have to happen.

In this chapter we provide students with exposure to kids in crisis. Worksheet themes include challenging issues such as teen suicide, handicapping conditions, living with terminal illness, family pressures, stress, and depression.

Keep in mind students' right for privacy when they are troubled. Sometimes they just need someone to listen; then there are times when a helping organization should step in. When problems are sealed from within, they often fester and grow worse.

Kids in trouble need to be aware that someone is out there for them—someone who cares and is willing to share.

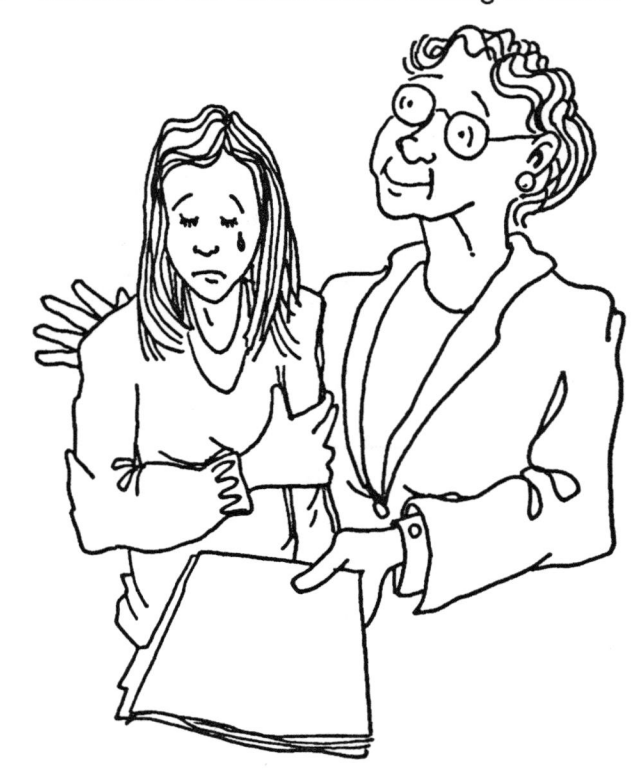

Hotline Available

SCENARIO

Wanda remembers Grannie telling her "worry is like a rocking chair; it gives you somethin' to do, but it don't get you anywhere." She wishes that she had Grannie around right now. She needs someone to talk to. She feels desperate.

The family is in a state of crisis; her parents fight all the time and she is depressed. Her troubles will not go away. She thought she could count on her boyfriend Jay, but they recently had a fight and he hit her. He said he didn't mean to and apologized, but she can't forget it. She is feeling crazy and can't concentrate on schoolwork. Should she call the Adolescent Suicide Hotline as she had seen advertised in her health book? Is there something she could do?

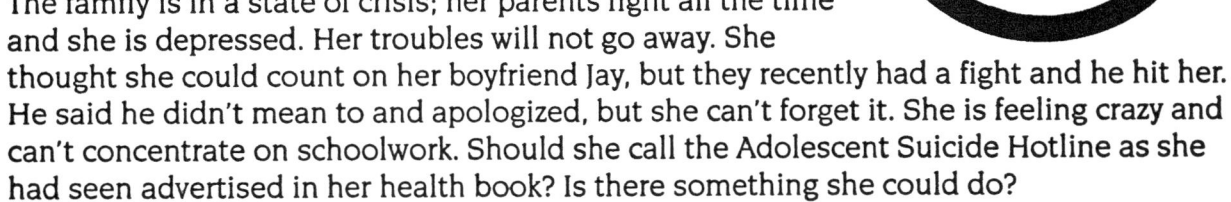

WHAT TO DO

You are Wanda's friend. Reach out a helping hand. How can you help her?

1. _____

2. _____

3. _____

4. _____

5. _____

Nikki's Story

SCENARIO

Nikki was a cool cheerleader and a good student. She belonged to lots of clubs and was a dependable member of the school newspaper. She was a friend to all who knew her.

During the summer between eighth and ninth grades, few friends saw Nikki, she seemed to be away a lot. Sometimes she was sick or just "not available."

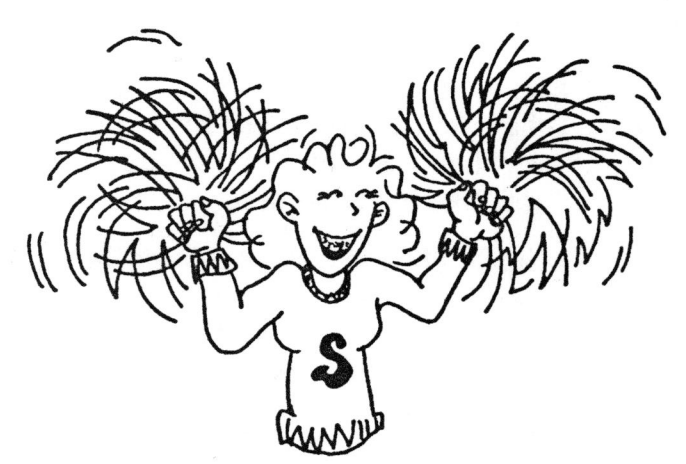

When school started in the fall Nikki seemed different. She was quiet and lacked her normal enthusiasm and zest for life. Concerned friends talked to the Physical Education teacher about their worries. (They knew they could trust her.) "She must be in some kind of trouble," they confided.

A month or so passed, then Mrs. Lewis, the school social worker, called four of Nikki's closest friends into her office. Nikki was there. "We have something private we would like to share with you girls," said Mrs. Lewis.

Nikki began to speak. "My parents do drugs," she said. "I was stressed out and felt that I had to keep it a secret and I thought that if I dropped my friends and school stuff, no one would find out. I didn't want anyone to know what was happening to my family. Then Mrs. Lewis helped me. She got me to go to Alateen and that's made a difference. It's helped me a lot and I don't feel embarrassed anymore."

"My Grandma and I got my folks in AA and we're going to be OK. More than ever, I need you to be my friends."

WHAT DO YOU THINK?

On the back of this page explain why support groups such as AA, Al-Anon, and Alateen work. (Do some research if you don't know.)

When you have a serious problem, how important is the support of good friends or a teacher you can trust?

_____

_____

Focus Word: **Alateen** — *A "spin-off" organization of Alcoholics Anonymous; a support group for teenagers.*

Plan To Be Happy

SCENARIO

When asked what her problem was, Lin Lang answered, "I'm adopted."

The girl was well loved and taken care of by her adoptive family, but she was curious about her origin and was uncomfortable about being different.

The guidance counselor asked Lin Lang to complete a plan. It helped her to focus on positive thoughts and see that she could be happy. She needed to work at it.

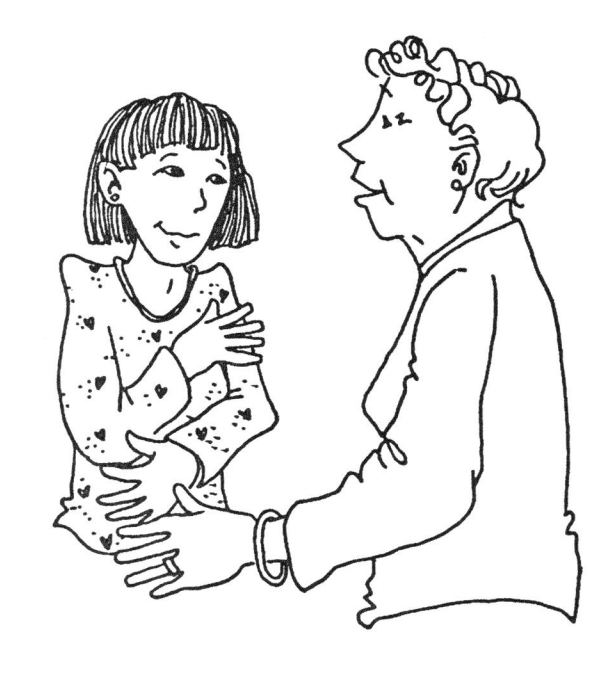

WHAT TO DO

Feeling down about something?

Tell about a time when you felt you weren't worth much. _____
_____
_____
_____
_____

Tell about a time when you felt like a million dollars. _____
_____
_____
_____
_____

What can you do to have more million dollar days? _____
_____
_____
_____
_____

Health and Success

Hassle Log

SCENARIO

Feeling tense and nervous? Are you mad at the world? Do you need something to help you keep tabs on anger?

This is it!

WHAT TO DO

Keep a record of provocative events; analyze the things that "trigger" stress in your life. Learn from your actions.

The day I got irritated

Place

Happening

What was said

What was done

How I felt afterward

What I wish I had done differently

How I kept my cool

Focus Word: **Provocation** — *Something that incites, instigates, angers, or irritates.*

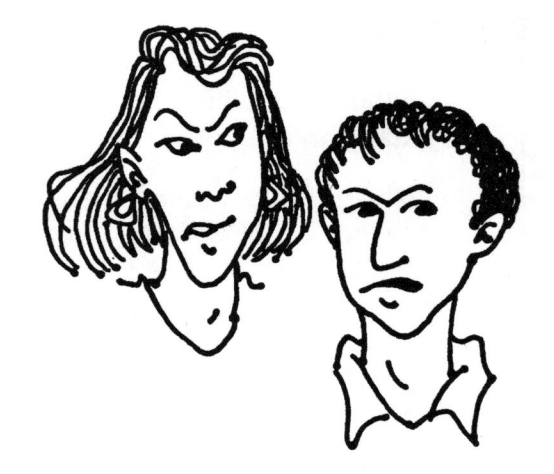

The Suicide

SCENARIO

Judy went to her brother's bedroom door one Saturday morning and called, "Hey, are you going to sleep all day?"

She discovered her twin brother with a plastic bag over his head. He was not breathing. The trauma that followed will last Judy a lifetime. There are so many unanswered questions for her and her family. Suicide is forever.

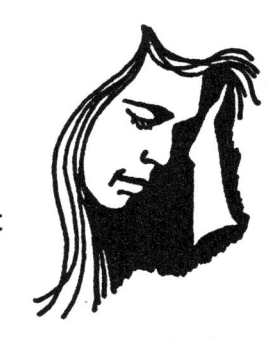

What happened to Jeff? The seventeen-year-old felt like a failure. His grandfather was a prominent attorney; his dad was a member of the firm. Both men were confident—and insisted—that the boy would one day join them. Jeff worked hard in school, but it was never good enough. He felt stupid and worthless.

Symptoms to be concerned about in a loved one:
- Depression
- Insomnia
- Chronic fatigue
- Drug abuse
- Alcohol use
- Outbursts of rage
- Feelings of sadness

A good way of heading off serious trouble is to get help at the first sign of trouble. Family crises are hard to handle.

IDEAS

Share your thinking with a friend. _____
_____
_____
_____
_____
_____

Focus Word: **Trauma** — *A startling experience which has a lasting effect on mental life.*

Be Someone Who Cares

SCENARIO

Jan became a statistic. Many people between the ages of 15 and 24 try to kill themselves each year. Many will try again. It's a sad—and very serious—problem.

Signs To Alert You—People who have suicidal tendencies may:

1. Say they want to die.
2. Start giving things away.
3. Abuse drugs or alcohol.
4. Display emotional highs or lows.
5. Withdraw from friends or family.
6. Become risk takers.

If you know someone with this type of behavior, what can you do? Don't be afraid to ask if you can help.

People like Jan need to know that someone cares. She survived her attempted suicide, but she may try again. If you were her friend, how would you reach out? What could you do or say?

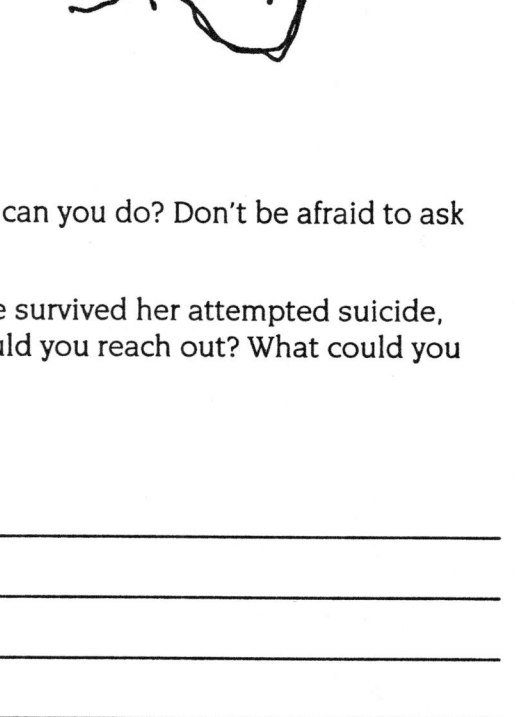

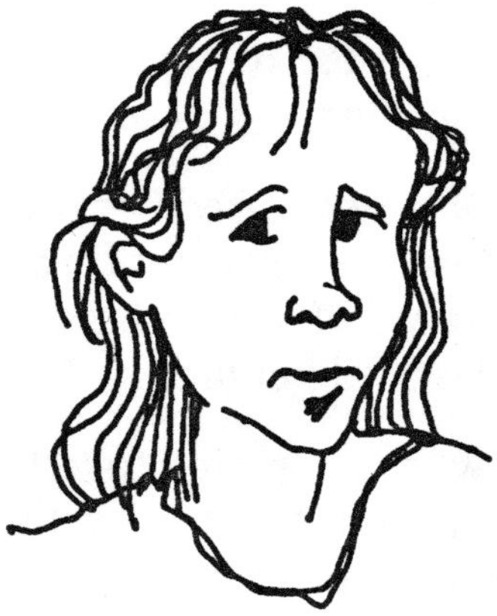

WRITE ABOUT IT

_____
_____
_____
_____
_____
_____
_____
_____
_____

Focus Word: **Negative risk taker** — *One who takes unnecessary chances that could be dangerous.*

No Bikini For Paula

SCENARIO

Paula's parents are obese. Every teen magazine she picks up emphasizes ultra-slim, pretty, young girls in bikinis. The most popular girls in school wear size sixes. When Paula reached a size fourteen, she decided it was time to do something drastic.

Today, the fifteen-year-old is plagued by the eating disorder anorexia. She has been hospitalized three times and may not be able to finish the school year with her classmates.

Stress is one of the leading causes of eating disorders. **Common stresses include:**
1. Feeling rejected; abandoned; alone.
2. Low self esteem; feeling like a failure.
3. Feeling ashamed.
4. Pressures at school, home or with friends.
5. Feelings of hopelessness or depression.
6. Sadness that won't go away.
7. Feeling afraid of someone or something.

WHAT DO YOU THINK?

Choose one or more of the suggested stressors that you think may have triggered Paula's problem. Explain your theory.

_____
_____
_____
_____
_____

Focus Word: **Anorexia Nervosa** — *An eating disorder disease, characterized by starvation and fear of food, that can ravage bodies and minds. It can be deadly, damaging vital parts of the body, including the heart.*

Getting Help

SCENARIO

Troubled? Frightened? Alone? Overwhelmed?

If you're bothered by a problem that won't go away, get help today. If a friend is in this situation, reach out a hand to help.

Adolescents are often faced with complicated problems that seem unsolvable. It's not easy being a teen; coping with pressures can be confusing. It is possible to get help to turn life around.

WHAT TO DO

The best sources of help are:
1. An adult you can trust
2. Counselor; teacher; school nurse
3. Police
4. Help hotline
5. Hospital
6. Minister; Priest; Rabbi

Where would you suggest your best friend get help if:
A. He has an abusive parent and is thinking of running away. _____
B. She thinks she might be pregnant. _____
C. A vicious street gang won't let him out. _____
D. She is doing drugs and can't function in school. _____
E. His girlfriend broke up with him and he can't handle it. _____
F. He has just found out he has HIV. _____

How important do you think a caring friend can be in time of crises? Explain.

_____
_____
_____
_____
_____

Focus Word: **Help Hotline** — *A 24-hour toll-free number provided by many organizations to provide immediate counseling or direction (your teacher might have a listing).*

Rate Your Life

SCENARIO

Do you wish you could be an Olympic athlete, look like Cindy Crawford or be smart enough to be the President?

How is your life? How happy are you to be where you are today? Place an "x" on the "life continuum."

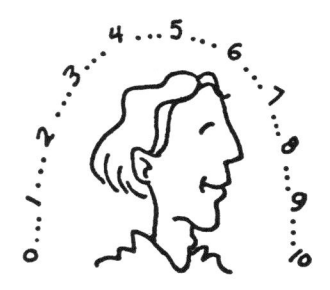

Life isn't so great "0"—1—2—3—4—5—6—7—8—9—"10" Life is great!

What about these kids?

Mike was born with cystic fibrosis, which is a hereditary lung disease. The fifteen-year-old must follow a daily routine of medication and physical therapy. (He takes 25 pills a day.)

Mike misses a lot of school because of time in the hospital. His disease will get worse unless they find a cure; heart-lung transplants are only temporary.

The boy has a good attitude about his terminal illness. And he's not alone. Many people with terminal diseases cope well with their illnesses. "I believe when people see me, they see someone who can be happy despite fighting against tremendous odds. I can inspire others," says Anne, who has a rare, immune disease called Wegener's Granulomatosis.

Beth broke a bone at the age of fourteen. The many tests that followed showed she has osteogenic sarcoma, a form of cancer that hits teenagers and people in their early twenties.

She has had surgery to remove a finger and her kneecap, and she faces more than a year of chemotherapy. The teenager is frequently in the hospital for other types of medical procedures and therapy.

"Having cancer is tough," she says, "but I'm learning to deal with it. I have to stick it out 'cause I believe I can survive."

WRITE ABOUT IT IT

Where do you think Michael, Anne, and Beth would put themselves on the continuum?

_____

_____

_____

Focus Word: **Life Continuum** — *A graphic representation showing a position between two extreme points.*

Health and Success

The Negative Chain

SCENARIO

You've heard the joke about the man who had a terrible day at work; he came home and yelled at his wife

    who spanked the kid
    who kicked the dog
    who bit the cat
    who ate the canary!

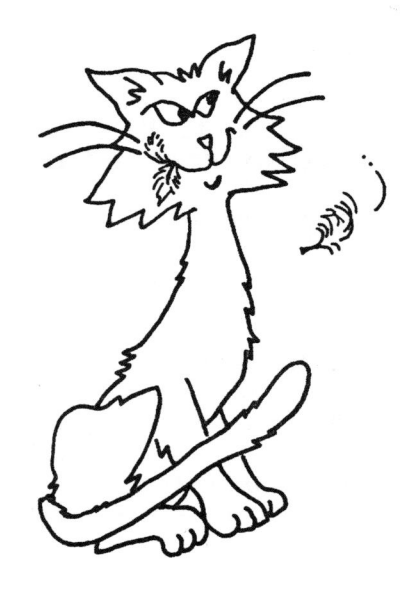

WRITE ABOUT IT

Briefly tell what could happen in each situation. Negative chains go on and on.

IF I get up late to finish homework THEN . . .
_____
_____
_____

IF I have a fight with my friend THEN . . .
_____
_____
_____

IF the principal calls my parents THEN . . .
_____
_____
_____

IF I cut class THEN . . .
_____
_____
_____

IF I forget to take my medicine THEN . . .
_____
_____
_____

IF I get mad at a teacher THEN . . .
_____
_____
_____

IF I get caught and get detention THEN . . .
_____
_____
_____

How far can this negative chain go? What then? _____
_____
_____

Focus Word: **Chain** — *Connected series of links which follow in succession.*

CHAPTER SIX

Natural Awakenings

74	**TEACHER'S PAGE**
75	*Serious Brain Activity* — Problem solving... Break It Down.
76	*Are You As Happy As Your Cat* — Gulliver's example... Can you follow it?
77	*Finding Out* — About mental health... How Smart Are You?
78	*Who Do You Know?* — Mental Health Models. How can you be like them?
79	*It's The Pits* — Three scenarios... How would you feel?
80	*The Sharper Image* — A research project... What did you learn?
81	*The Attitude Adjustment* — Jeeper's scenario... Problem's sources.
82	*Better Than Best* — Room for improvement. How can you accomplish more?
83	*A Do-It-Yourself Job* — Words of wisdom... What do you think?
84	*Accentuate The Positive* — Count your blessings. Your life is great!
86	*Magnificent Or Mediocre* — Evaluate... Who are you?
87	*Tell It Like It Is* — Three kids... Help them out!
88	*Can-Do Plan* — How to get out! A good exercise.
89	*Make It Happen* — What are your aspirations? Start with one out of sight!

Health and Success

Healthy Ways—Healthy Days

While it is important to respect the amazing human machine—the body—it's equally important to work toward good mental health; you cannot separate the two.

In the early adolescent years it's crucial for youngsters to gain an awareness of what makes them think, feel and react the way they do. Activities provided are based upon everyday dilemmas that may trouble them or their peers, and suggest ways to handle these situations by focusing on their own lives.

Techniques for critical thinking and problem solving can help students internalize their management skills.

An independent thinking and writing exercise by "pair-sharing" or small-group work is suggested. Kids need to know that they are not alone; strong human relationships can evolve to enhance the subject matter.

Good health is a never-ending process; it must last a lifetime!

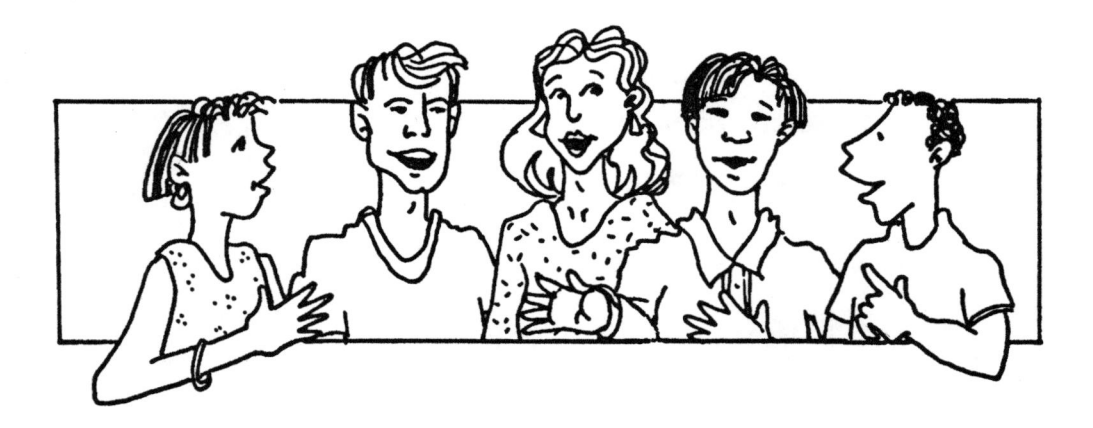

Serious Brain Activity

SCENARIO

As you grow older, you begin to understand what makes you tick—why you think and act the way you do.

Good mental health will help you work though problems and pressures you may feel. The way you face the day-to-day difficult problems is important.

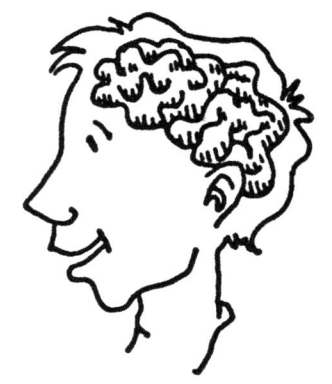

WHAT TO DO

Here's A Groaner

Think about a problem you have had; a failure or disappointment. You felt _____

_____

_____

How did you handle the situation? _____

_____

_____

An option might be _____

_____

_____

Share the situation with a classmate. Discuss other options together.

Now I think _____

_____

_____

_____

_____

Focus Word: **Mental Health** — *A condition of the mind with reference to soundness and vigor.*

Are You As Happy As Your Cat?

SCENARIO

The minute Marcia's cat Gulliver was let out of the house he got into a vicious fight with the neighbor's dog, Thor. Gulliver and Thor hate each other.

Minutes later Gulliver came back into the house. He jumped up on Marcia's lap, purred loudly, got comfy, and went to sleep.

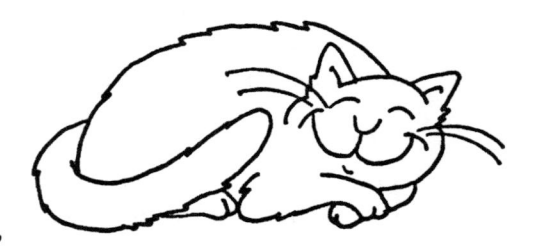

Marcia thought about the fight she had with her mom that morning before school. It was really bad. She's still furious that her mom won't let her see a movie because—in Mom's words—"It's too mature." Lots of kids are going.

Marcia didn't like feeling this way. "Why can't I be more like Gulliver?" she thought.

WHAT DO YOU THINK?

Should I sneak to the movies? _____

_____

_____

_____

Should I try to talk to my Mom again? What could I say? _____

_____

_____

_____

_____

How can I handle my anger? _____

_____

_____

_____

_____

Focus Word: **Mature** — *Grown-up; adult.*

Finding Out

WHAT DO YOU THINK?

How Smart Are You?

1. What do we mean by mental health?
   _____
   _____

2. What are some characteristics mentally healthy people often have?
   _____

3. What's a good thing to do when a problem troubles you?
   _____
   _____
   _____

4. Why is good mental health important?
   _____
   _____
   _____

5. Why is it generally a good idea to talk over a problem with someone you can trust?
   _____
   _____
   _____

6. Go over your answers with a classmate. Discuss your thinking.

   I learned (re-learned) _____
   _____
   _____

Focus Word: **Characteristic**— *A distinctive or typical quality; a manner.*

Who Do You Know?

WHAT DO YOU THINK?

The following are characteristics of individuals with good mental health. At the end of each description, write the names (or initials) of people you know who "fit the bill."

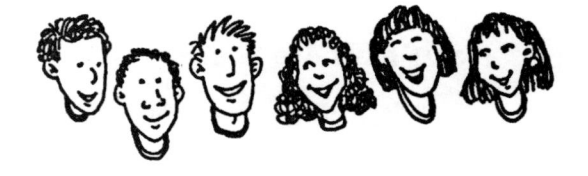

1. They generally feel comfortable with themselves _____
2. They can handle life's disappointments _____
3. They have self respect _____
4. They give love to others _____
5. They are considerate of others _____
6. They try to understand viewpoints other than their own _____
7. They don't push people around _____
8. They accept responsibility _____
9. They have goals and plan ahead _____
10. They do something about their problems _____
11. They are not "hot heads" _____
12. They can be trusted _____

Circle the numbers you think also describe you.

Place an "X" beside one of the characteristics you need to work on.

Room for improvement? I can begin by _____
_____
_____
_____
_____

Focus Word: **Hot Head** — *A person who jumps to conclusions or gets angry quickly.*

It's The Pits!

WHAT DO YOU THINK?

One of the keys to working with and understanding others, is to put yourself in his or her place. How would you feel if you were in the place of . . .

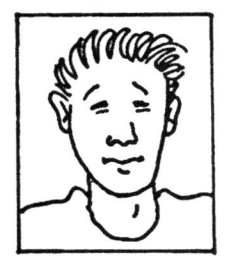

Ray was in an automobile accident that seemed like a never-ending nightmare. Kevin had been drinking and was driving the car. Kevin was killed.

Ray has no recollection of the fatal accident, but knows he faces months of hospitalization and therapy for his broken back. His friend Alex was in the car also, but was uninjured. Alex cries a lot.

_____

_____

_____

Suzi was always cool and confident until she fell in love with Todd. (Her mom said it was just a crush.) She did some things she now knows she should not have done, and feels embarrassed and hurt. Todd has just dropped her and is dating her old friend Jamie.

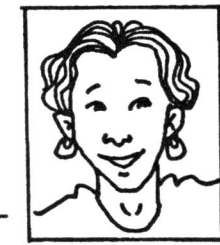

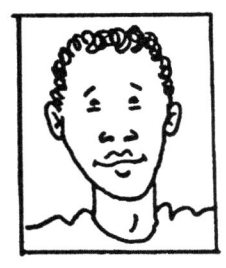

_____

_____

_____

Dex was the lead singer for a school rock band, "Hi Jinx." He was pretty good and the kids all liked his style. As the band became more popular, a few of the members started doing drugs. One night Dex complained to some of the guys that they weren't playing as well as they once did. He believes drug use is wrong. The next day the other members told Dex they had a replacement for him. They said Dex was a "prima donna" and too hard to get along with.

_____

_____

_____

Sometimes we get discouraged by a sudden turn of events in our lives and find it hard to understand. It's important to think things out slowly and work them out—the best for each of us—one day at a time.

Take life's disappointments in stride!

The Sharper Image

SCENARIO

Mental health isn't something we achieve as adults. It's never finished and over with at any stage of life. We can always improve on our life and make it better. We keep growing!

Choose a popular personality or historical figure. Search for current information (or historical data) that tells something about that person. Do some analysis and decide what kind of person he or she really is or was. Search for evidence of characteristics such as kindness, humility, empathy, warmth, stability and responsibility.

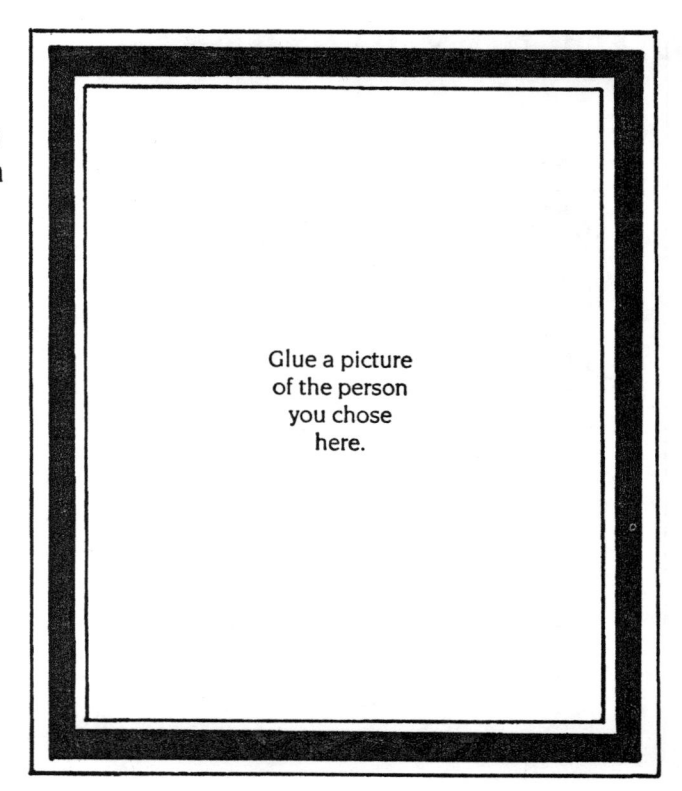

Glue a picture of the person you chose here.

WRITE ABOUT IT

Get that sharper image. Is it the way you thought it would be?

I chose _____

Because _____

She or he is or was _____

_____

I think she or he is or was _____

_____

_____

I learned _____

_____

_____

Focus Word: **Personality** — *A distinctive or notable character.*

The Attitude Adjustment

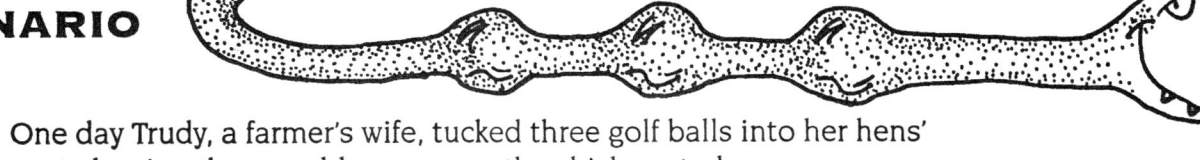

SCENARIO

One day Trudy, a farmer's wife, tucked three golf balls into her hens' nests hoping they would encourage the chickens to lay more eggs.

A few days later she noticed that the "phony eggs" had vanished. She mentioned the missing golf balls to her husband; it was a mystery to both.

The next day, son Tim was concerned when he spotted his pet snake Jeepers lying stretched out, not in its usual sleeping coil. The reptile seemed lethargic. The boy really began to worry when he saw three large lumps in the middle of the four foot, black, rat snake.

It seems the snake had been robbing the hens' nests, and . . . you guessed it.

A veterinarian surgically removed the golf balls from the snake. Jeepers had an instant "attitude adjustment!" True story!

It's tough for those of us who have attitude problems. We can't have them surgically removed.

Some of the things that may be a source of anger, or "attitude problem" are:
- Parents embarrassing kids in front of friends
- Teachers who give unexpected grades or tests
- Friends for not agreeing with them
- Siblings (for existing)
- Fight with a boy or girlfriend
- Gang pressure
- Frustrations with being a teen

WRITE ABOUT IT

How do you know when you need an attitude adjustment? _____

_____

Maybe I could _____

_____

Focus Word: **Attitude** — *Position, disposition, or manner with regard to a person or thing.*

Health and Success

Better Than Best

SCENARIO

"If you are content with the best you have done, you will never do the best you can do!"

Advances in medicine and technology would not be where they are today if we settled for the best we have done. Mistakes and failures happen to all of us. But we can learn from our errors and become less likely to make the same errors again.

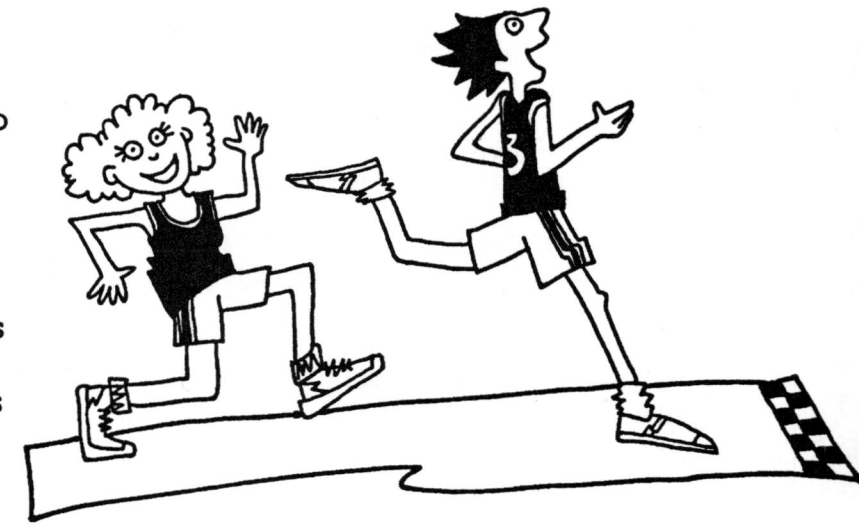

WRITE ABOUT IT

List some things you have accomplished and feel good about:

1. _____
2. _____
3. _____

Congratulations! You're great! What are some things you can do better if you work harder?

1. _____
2. _____
3. _____

Starting tomorrow you could _____
_____
_____
_____

Focus Word: **Accomplishment** — *To bring to pass; carry out; perform.*

A Do-It-Yourself Job

SCENARIO

"Life is a do-it-yourself job!"

The gaudy, purple and orange poster bearing this message hangs in the office of Mrs. Owens, the school social worker.

Kids walk in daily with problems ranging from school failure to parental abuse. Some are victims of hate and intolerance; they have suffered crimes of the body, the mind, and the heart.

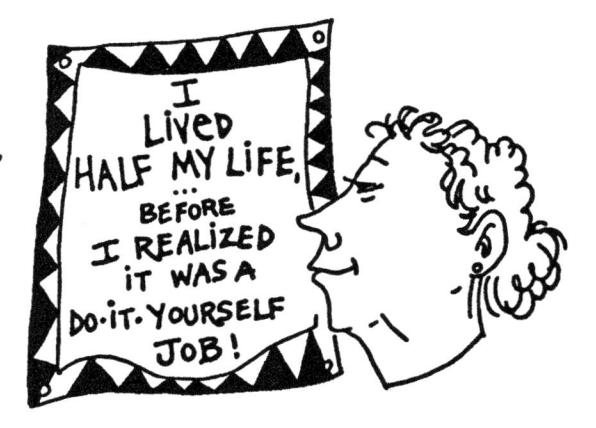

Mrs. Owens provides needed support while piecing broken lives back together (with the help of the significant words on the poster). What do you think they mean? How can they provide a positive message for you or someone you know?

WRITE ABOUT IT

I think _____

_____

_____

_____

Copy the words from the poster in the space below. Cut them out. Give it to someone or post it where you will see it as a reminder.

Focus Word: **Do-It-Yourself Job** — *Working it out; taking control and responsibility.*

Accentuate The Positive

SCENARIO

You have forty-eight hours to enjoy. Take notes on all the positive things that happened to you during those hours.

WRITE ABOUT IT

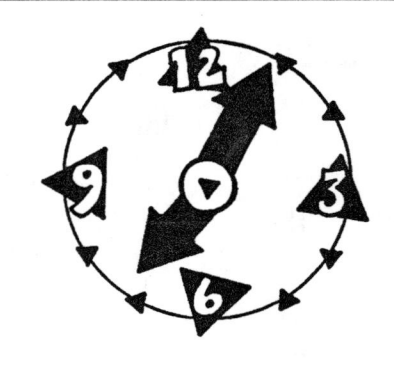

Day One

AM	PM
People	People
Places	Places
Things	Things
Good Stuff	Good Stuff

The best part of the day was _____
_____
_____
_____

Day Two

	AM	PM
	People	People
	Places	Places
	Things	Things
	Good Stuff	Good Stuff

The best part of the day was _____

_____

_____

_____

_____

_____

_____

Focus Word: **Positive** — *A good quality; the opposite of negative.*

Health and Success

Magnificent Or Mediocre

SCENARIO

Good things seldom just drop out of the sky; we make them happen!

Why settle for a mediocre life when with some work and determination you can have a magnificent life? How positive is your personality? An upbeat personality is a plus!

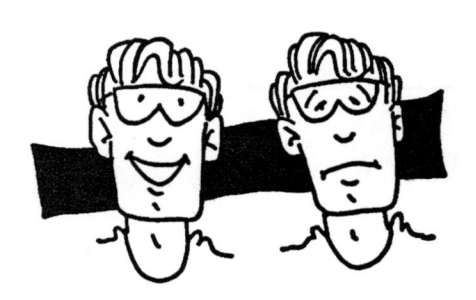

WHAT DO YOU THINK?

Look at the following statements and identify each with a "P" or an "N" (Positive/Negative)

_____ I am happy most of the time

_____ I'm often tired

_____ I feel good about myself

_____ I don't like myself

_____ I like to try new things

_____ I like other people

_____ I like being alone a lot

_____ I'm sort of lazy

_____ I'm afraid to try new things

_____ I feel angry a lot

_____ I have a lot of energy

_____ I work hard

_____ I reach out and help others

_____ I feel healthy

Which three do you think best describe you and why?

1. _____
2. _____
3. _____

Is there a character trait you could work on? _____

_____

_____

Get Going—You can be magnificent!

Focus Word: **Mediocre** — *Of only moderate quality; neither good nor bad; OK.*

Tell It Like It Is

SCENARIO

React to the following scenarios with a partner. What is wrong with each? Give each kid a message.

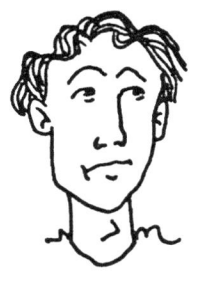

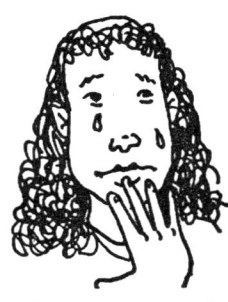

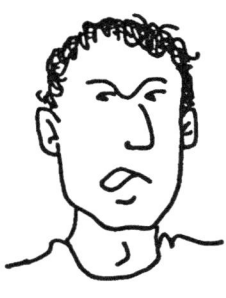

When Amid gets back a test paper with a poor grade on it, he tears it up and throws it away before he checks the mistakes.

_____
_____

Roxie starts crying whenever her Dad reprimands her. She knows he can't stand tears and he will leave her alone if she cries.

_____
_____

Ian is big and bossy. He's a tough football player and always pushes around the small, smart kids. He calls them "geeks."

_____
_____

WHAT DO YOU THINK?

A mentally healthy person accepts his or her own shortcomings and tries to do something about them!

_____
_____

Focus Word: **Shortcomings** — *Failures or defects in conduct or condition.*

Can-Do Plan

SCENARIO

"I hate my life!"

"I'm in a rut!"

"Why me?"

"I can't."

"I shouldn't have."

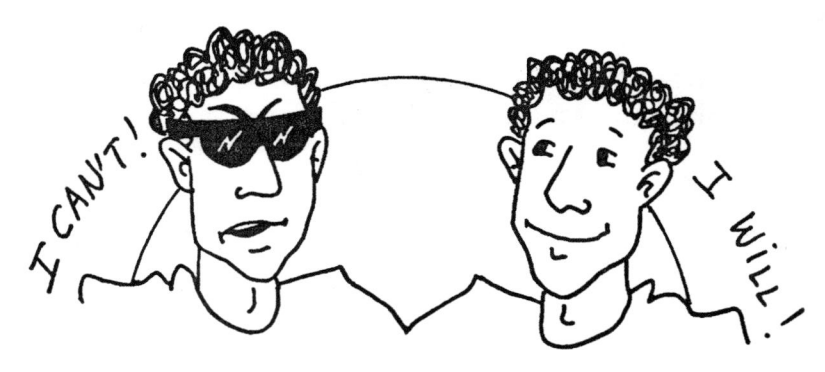

Take off the dark sunglasses and start looking for a way to get out of that bad situation! Remember, in most cases you alone are not responsible for the negative things happening in your life.

WHAT DO YOU THINK?

Start with this simple "exercise." It's easy and anyone can do it.

Can-DO Plan

Problems—

Possible cause—

Effect on me—

Can do this—

Or, **can** do this—

Will do this!—

Focus Word: **Exercise** — *A procedure; to put into action.*

Make It Happen

SCENARIO

Without personal motivation we can't take that first step to make special things happen.

WRITE ABOUT IT

Respond to the following:

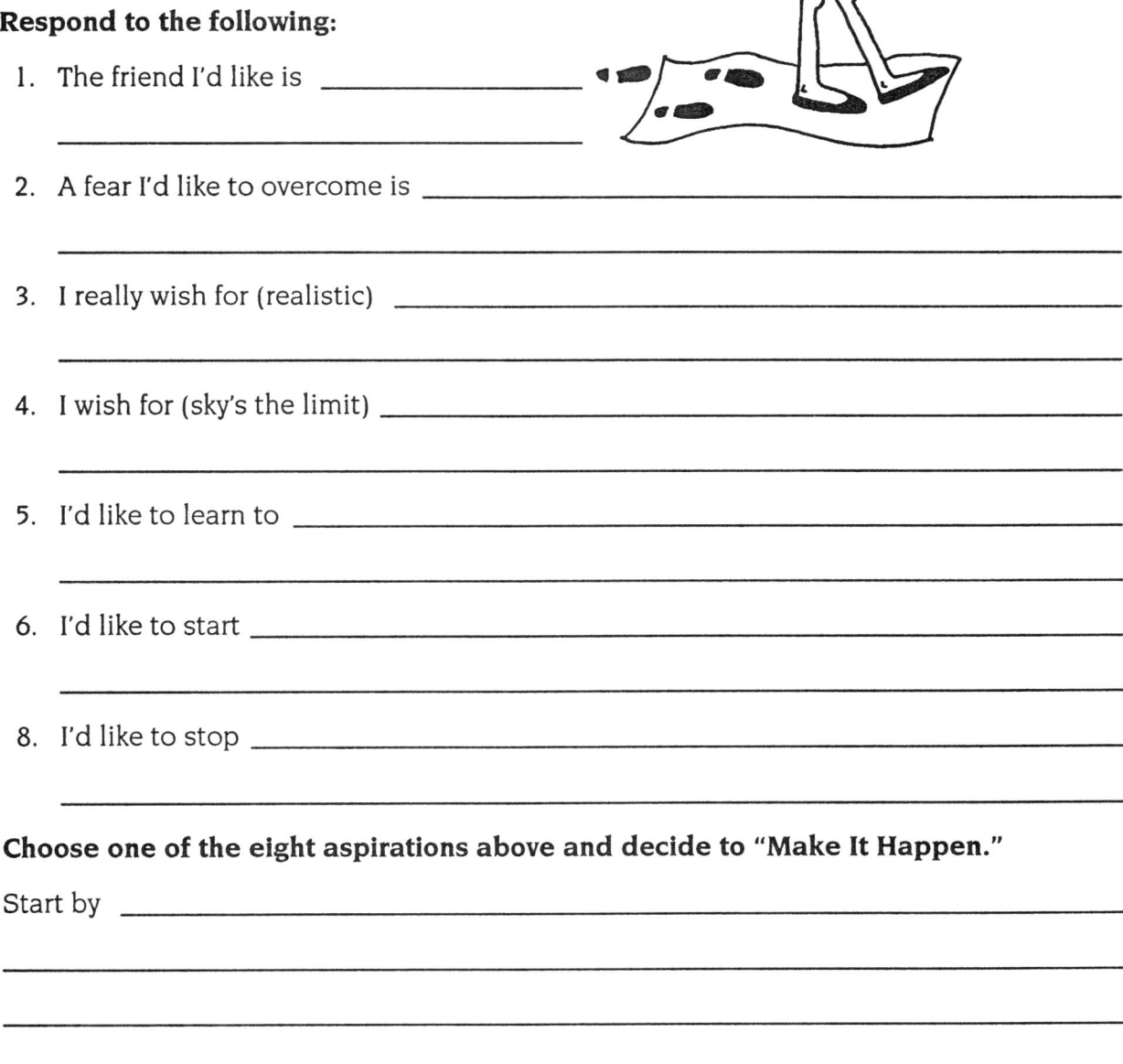

1. The friend I'd like is _____
_____

2. A fear I'd like to overcome is _____
_____

3. I really wish for (realistic) _____
_____

4. I wish for (sky's the limit) _____
_____

5. I'd like to learn to _____
_____

6. I'd like to start _____
_____

8. I'd like to stop _____
_____

Choose one of the eight aspirations above and decide to "Make It Happen."

Start by _____
_____
_____
_____

Focus Word: **Motivation** — *Something that promotes a person to act in a certain way; incentive.*

APPENDIX

Briefly

In this chapter are provided bits and pieces of information.

The student inventory "Getting To Know You" can be an important tool in working with young teens. When honesty and confidentiality are stressed, students usually show insight into what makes each other tick. By stressing confidentiality, you also reinforce your concern about students' privacy and your care for them.

Notes, letters, or monthly newsletters can focus on the important issues of the times. Try to avoid dwelling on the negative aspects of our "uncivilized world;" be helpful, emphasizing the positive whenever possible. The letter suggested in this chapter may be personalized with names and events for added relevance.

The section "Getting Help" is a very brief listing of the helping organizations that are available for the most frequent—and often complex—teen difficulties. Other school personnel, local library or telephone directory can provide you with many others. Teenagers must know that there is someplace to turn when they think a problem is too big to be solved.

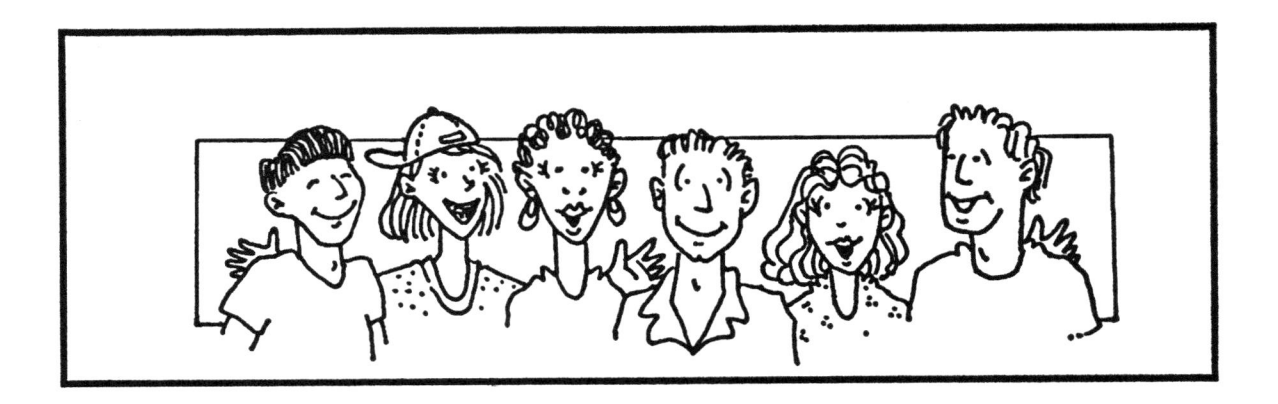

Marijuana Alert

Abuse that may last a lifetime could begin during the early teen years. Marijuana is often the first illegal substance your students may experiment with. Smoking among high school students has jumped sharply.

Young people think that smoking pot is not a big deal—it can't hurt them. However, because of a new method of processing and harvesting plants, it is now about twenty times more potent than in the sixties and seventies.

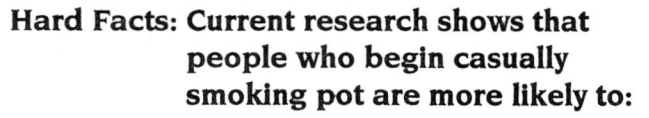

Hard Facts: Current research shows that people who begin casually smoking pot are more likely to:
1. Move on to hard drugs such as cocaine
2. Become victims of teen violence
3. Resort to crime to obtain drug money
4. Damage long and short term memory, lungs, and immune system
5. Have unsafe sex and transmit HIV
6. Develop lung cancer

Side Effects: Smoking pot may seem like fun and may seem to promote "bonding," but some frightening side effects are:
1. Depression and mood swings
2. Apathy and introversion; lack of motivation
3. Paranoia and nervousness
4. Isolation
5. Suicide

The Warning: Talking to students about concepts such as breaking the law and addiction are not enough. Students must be informed of all issues that surround pot smoking because their future health and wellness are at stake. Leaving a "marijuana alert" up to the drug counselors may be too little too late!

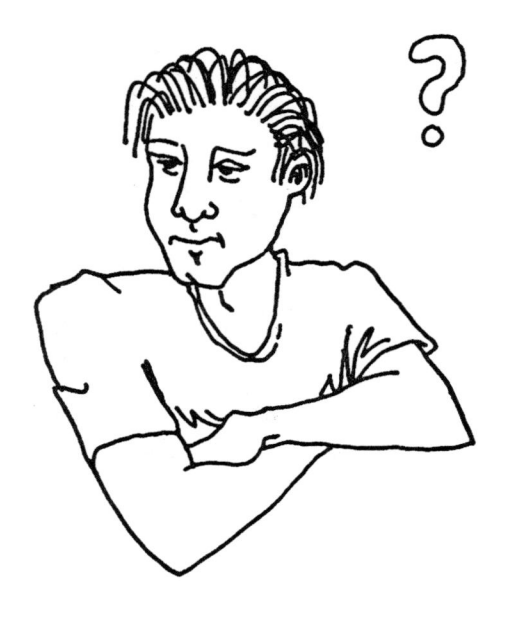

Health Briefs

Peruse newspapers and magazines for current health and fitness advice, discoveries and emerging trends. Make it a "daily quest." Be alert! For example:

Binge and Purge — Teens who have chronic illnesses such as diabetes and asthma are more likely to be dissatisfied with their bodies and develop eating disorders.

Couch Spuds — Many adults don't engage in any physical activity during their leisure time. Begin now with an "attitude adjustment" to avoid the risk of heart disease and other ailments in the future.

Risk of AIDS — Teens make up about one quarter of the newly infected AIDS victims. Prevention programs must begin early.

Fight the Microbes — New bugs are emerging and old ones are making a comeback! We live in an environment in which diseases can spread anywhere around the world. One of the dangers is the overuse of antibiotics, which in some cases have caused drug-resistant bacteria to evolve.

Asthma — This disease has emerged as a special problem among inner-city kids. Factors such as air pollution and living conditions—cockroaches, mice, rats, cats, and cigarette smoke—are some of the villains.

Hope — There is hope for those living with HIV. A new class of drugs has raised hopes that infection could become a livable—but chronic—condition.

Increasing Problem — "Gateway Drugs" are those usually tried first by children: tobacco, alcohol, marijuana and inhalants.

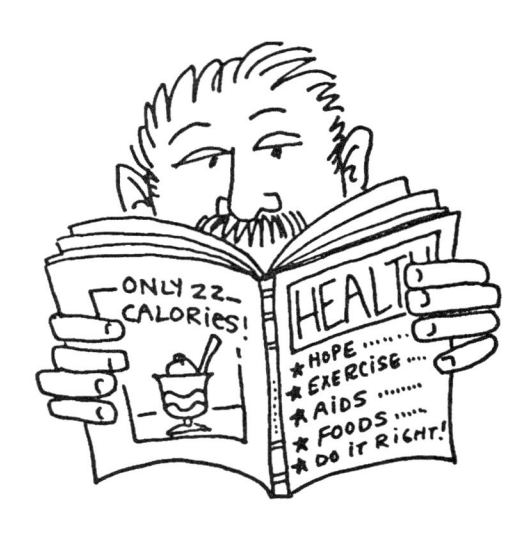

Don't Go To Pot

Teaching children to "say no" is not solely the job of teachers or counselors. To maintain a continuity of effort, parents must become a crucial link.

The following text, when sent home by a teacher, may foster a greater degree of involvement on the part of the adult caregiver.

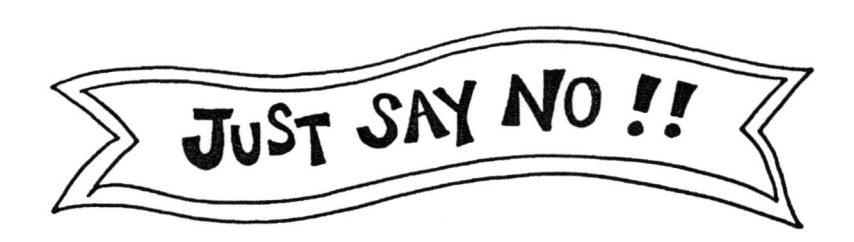

JUST SAY NO !!

Dear_____,

Your child has arrived at the age of experimentation. This is perhaps the most important time for parents to focus on drug prevention.

These are the years when crucial decisions about the use of alcohol and **drugs may** first be made. "Gateway drugs"—tobacco, alcohol, marijuana and inhalants—are generally the first tried. However, they can create a dependency that can last a lifetime.

The following suggestions may be practiced with your child to help make appropriate choices:

- Say "No"—no discussion; don't argue; be firm. Say "No" and show you mean it.

- Give reason—I don't do that; I'm busy; sorry, not interested.

- Suggest other things—a movie; a game; a project. Reject the activity, **not the friend.**

- Leave—When all else fails, and the above suggestions don't work, remove yourself from the situation immediately. Join another group, go home, or go to class.

Communicate often with your children. Counteract peer influence with **parental** influence.

Send a clear message—you love them and don't want them to "go to pot."

Sincerely,

Getting Help

The following helping organizations are available for the most common and complex problems. Updated information may be obtained yearly from the *Directory of National Hotlines*, which may be found in the Dewey Decimal System under number 361–323.

Abuse—Physical, Mental, Verbal, Sexual.

CHILDHELP USA
6463 Independence Ave.
Woodland Hills, CA 91367
A nonprofit charity combating child abuse.
(818) 347-7280

PARENTS ANONYMOUS
675 W Foothill Blvd, Suite 220
Claremont, CA 91711-3475
An international self-help organization for parents.
(909) 621-6184

Adoption—For adoptees who have problems

ALMA SOCIETY
Adoptee's Liberty Movement Assn.
PO Box 727 Radio City Station
New York, NY 10033
Facilitates reunions of children and natural parents
(212) 581-1568

ADOPTIVE FAMILIES OF AMERICA
2309 Como Ave.
Minneapolis, MN 55108
Provides support and information for people in adoptive families.

Substance Abuse

JUST SAY NO HOTLINE
National Clearinghouse for Alcohol and Drug Information
2101 Webster St, Suite 1300
Oakland, CA 94612
(800) 729-6686

Getting Help (cont.)

Eating Disorders—Anorexia Nervosa, Bulimia, overeating and compulsive dieting

OVEREATERS ANONYMOUS
Self-Help World Service Organization
PO Box 92870
Los Angeles, CA 90009
(213) 542-8363

AMERICAN ANOREXIA/BULIMIA ASSOCIATION
165 W 46th St, #1108
New York, NY 10036
(212) 575-6200

Family Crises—Coping with death, disease, accident, dissension, or financial

AL-ANON FAMILY/ALATEEN
Group Headquarters
1600 Corporate Landing Pkwy
Virginia Beach, VA 23454-5617
Self-help fellowship of families of alcoholics; Alateen for teens
1-(800) 356-9996

COMPASSIONATE FRIENDS
Box 3696
Oak Brook, IL 60522-3696
For parents and siblings of a child who has died.
(312) 990-0010

FAMILY SERVICE AMERICA
1700 W. Lake Park Drive
Milwaukee, WI 53224
Family Counseling and referral
(800) 221-2681

STEPFAMILY ASSOCIATION OF AMERICA
650 J St, Suite 1205
Lincoln, NE 68508
Sponsors gatherings and distributes materials.
(800) 735-0329

Mental Health

NATIONAL MENTAL HEALTH ASSOCIATION
Provides free information on a variety of health topics
1-(800) 969-6642

NATIONAL RUNAWAYS SWITCHBOARD
Provides 24-hour operator crisis counseling to handle situations of imminent danger; has shelters and referrals available.
1-(800) 621-4000